Akponne Tiamiou

# African alternative medicine: our culture, our future

Akponne Tiamiou

# African alternative medicine: our culture, our future

ScienciaScripts

**Imprint**



Cover image: www.ingimage.com

This book is a translation from the original published under ISBN 978-613-8-43161-9.

Publisher:
Sciencia Scripts
is a trademark of
Dodo Books Indian Ocean Ltd. and OmniScriptum S.R.L publishing group

120 High Road, East Finchley, London, N2 9ED, United Kingdom
Str. Armeneasca 28/1, office 1, Chisinau MD-2012, Republic of Moldova, Europe
Printed at: see last page
**ISBN: 978-620-6-25768-4**

Table of contents :

Part 1 5

Chapter 1 5

Chapter 2 25

Part 2 40

Chapter 3 40

Chapter 4 60

Chapter 5 64

Part 3 81

Chapter 6 81

Chapter 7 89

# GENERAL INTRODUCTION

Since the dawn of mankind, we have always sought to preserve our health. To achieve this, he uses the resources of his environment. He has always adopted behaviours and practices based on his perception of things and on the socio-cultural and socio-religious model of his environment and time.

Plant, animal and mineral species are the main natural resources used by man for protection, disease prevention and treatment, and health rehabilitation.

In Africa, as elsewhere, these resources have been used for ages by traditional practitioners who acquired their knowledge and know-how through observation, spiritual revelation, personal experience, training and direct information from their predecessors (DANNERMANN R, 1982).

Traditional medicine, rich in diversity, reflects the therapeutic richness of the continent's cultural heritage. Indeed, African flora in general, and Beninese flora in particular, still contains many plant species that have not been identified by biologists, and whose therapeutic virtues are perhaps still unknown.

Faced with the emergence of a number of chronic diseases such as tuberculosis, diabetes, sickle cell anemia, HIV/AIDS and other infectious diseases, the healthcare system based on the Western model is proving increasingly inadequate for the comprehensive management of illnesses.

In fact, "everyone agrees today that modern medicine is failing to deliver all the results expected of it. Worse still, it is becoming increasingly alienating and impoverishing" (OUINSOU S. E, 1994).

Statistics from the World Health Organization (WHO) estimate that over 80% of Benin's population use traditional medicine as their first line of health care.

Traditional medicine is very popular. It is generally when this fails that patients turn to modern medicine.

However, there are cases where traditional medicine has succeeded where modern medicine has failed. There are many examples of this in the case of psychiatric disorders.

Despite the importance of traditional medicine within national communities, particularly in rural areas, it remains outside the official health system in Benin.

If traditional medicine is to be put to the best possible use in the official health system, more attention needs to be paid to it.

The aim of this study is to examine the various ways in which traditional medicine has been integrated into the official health system in Benin.

This overall objective is broken down into five(05) specific objectives:

- research the foundations of traditional medicine ;
- study the basics of traditional medical practice ;
- examine the framework for collaboration between traditional medicine practitioners and health workers;
- identify the illnesses treated by traditional healers and list some of the remedies they use;
- Finally, to assess the safety aspects of traditional health care offerings in terms of efficacy, safety and quality.

To conduct this study, a number of hypotheses were put forward:

- **First hypothesis**: Traditional medicine practices are based on the socio-cultural and sometimes religious determinants of communities (convents are veritable schools where the practice of traditional medicine and pharmacopoeia are taught);
- **Second hypothesis**: The techniques used by traditional healers in the practice of their arts are based on their long experience acquired and passed down from generation to generation.
- **Third hypothesis**: Collaboration between traditional healers and conventional medical practitioners is not always straightforward;
- **Fourth hypothesis**: In addition to the supernatural illnesses referred to them, tradipraticians also offer care for common pathologies encountered during consultations in conventional health facilities;
- **Fifth hypothesis**: The efficacy, safety and quality of the care offered by traditional healers in the management of illnesses are evidenced by the patient's recovery or relief.

At the end of the study, the following results are expected:

- The socio-cultural and religious foundations of traditional medicine are justified;
- The technical basis of traditional medicine practices is well known;
- Collaboration between tradipraticians and health-care workers is analyzed. The pathologies treated by tradipraticians are identified, some of the plants used are listed and six of them have been subjected to biological testing (phytochemical screening and toxicity);
- Patients treated by traditional healers we met testified to having been cured or relieved.

This research was carried out using a two-stage methodological approach:

- The first stage was the literature search. This decisive step enabled us to gather and consult many valuable sources of information to better define the research problem.

This stage was also decisive in the development of instruments for collecting information in the field, and helped to set the objectives of the study and develop the research hypotheses accordingly.

- The second, exciting stage is the field survey.

And as Beau and Weber, paraphrased by HOUINGNIHIN R.A. (2005), put it: "Fieldwork means wanting to connect with the facts, to talk with respondents, to better understand individuals and social processes. Without this thirst for discovery, without this desire to know, almost to do battle, fieldwork becomes a formality, an academic exercise, flat and uninteresting".

The fieldwork stage was used to gather information on all aspects of the practice of traditional medicine in Benin. Above all, it gave us the opportunity to share and exchange views on a wide range of traditional medicine experiences.

All the information gathered in the field has been carefully processed and analyzed to make the best use of it.

Qualitative information was processed manually, while quantitative data was processed by computer.

This study is divided into three main parts:

- The first part is devoted to a review of the literature and a methodological approach;
- The second part presents the results of our research;
- The third part provides a critical analysis of the results obtained, without calling into question the research findings. It explores other modalities for the judicious integration of Traditional Medicine into the official health care system in Benin.

# PART ONE :

# METHODOLOGICAL APPROACH

## CHAPTER 1$^{ER}$ : LITERATURE REVIEW

### A- Concepts of Traditional Medicine and Pharmacopoeia

### 1- Traditional Medicine and Pharmacopoeia

#### a) Traditional Medicine

A group of experts from the World Health Organization (WHO), meeting from February 9 to 13, 1976, defined Traditional Medicine as "all knowledge and practices, whether explicable or not, for diagnosing, preventing or eliminating physical, mental or social imbalance, based exclusively on experience and observation handed down from generation to generation, orally or in writing" (WHO, 1976).

But in 1991, in his thesis on pharmacy, NATABOU D.F. pointed out that medicine is not static. It evolves, and its evolution inevitably results in a medical system that is different from what it was at the outset and from what it will be in the future.

Abagomi SOFOWORA (1996)[1] Nigerian author, offers a neutral yet open definition: "Traditional Medicine can be defined as the overall combination of knowledge and practices, whether explicable or not, used to diagnose, prevent or eliminate physical, mental or social illness, and which may be based exclusively on ancient experience and observations handed down from generation to generation, orally or in writing".

The author adds: "In Africa, this definition can be broadened", and adds a sentence along the following lines: "Taking into account the original concept of nature, which includes the material world, the sociological environment, whether living or dead, and the metaphysical forces of the universe".

Abagomi SOFOWORA(1996) first emphasizes the generational aspect of Traditional Medicine knowledge: "This is knowledge acquired through experience, and passed on to the next generation of healers, during their initiation, for centuries. Transmission is generally oral. He goes on to stress the importance of understanding the **socio-cultural** context of these healing practices.

He also emphasized the sociological environment, whether "living or dead". By this we mean the power of ancestors who have disappeared, or of neighbors or acquaintances who are often ill-intentioned and can affect the physical and psychological balance of the living, leading to recourse to the healer for traditional treatment.

Finally, the author speaks of "metaphysical forces of the universe". By this we mean the spirits and divinities that influence the equilibrium of the living.

The practitioner of Traditional Medicine was defined by a regional committee of the

WHO Office for Africa (1976) as a person recognized by the community in which he or she lives as competent to provide health care using plant, animal and mineral substances or other methods.

These methods are based on social, cultural and religious elements as well as on the knowledge, attitudes and beliefs prevalent in the community about physical, mental and social well-being and the causes of illness and disability" (Sofowora 1982). This definition has been long and widely used.

Traditional medicine is not only concerned with the biological aspect of patients' ailments, but also with a nosology and etiology that call upon the physical context of life, but also the spiritual context (divinities, ancestors) and the social context (family and neighbors).

Illness is seen not only as a physical imbalance, but also as a social and spiritual one that needs to be treated simultaneously.

David T. OKPAKO of the University of Ibadan in Nigeria, in turn characterizes Traditional Medicine by three major paradigms:

- the cause of the disease may be supranatural;
- the diagnosis of the condition can be made by divination;
- treatment of illness requires a message, a ritual of preparation using plant, animal or mineral substances (OKPAKO D. 1999).
- The plant, animal or mineral preparations used serve as "medicine", and can sometimes have spiritual roles.

As far back as the 10th and 11th centuries, the Yoruba knew and practiced traditional medicine. One of the most beautiful pages in the history of these peoples teaches that a woman named OBATALA, an important character among the many children of the ancestor ODUDUA, knew how to treat illnesses by prescribing leaves and roots for infusions and poultices. She also helped pregnant women give birth (YARI B. J. 2008).

Having attempted to define the concept of traditional medicine, what can we say about the concept of traditional pharmacopoeia?

**b) Traditional Pharmacopoeia**

In the reference framework for harmonization of registration procedures for medicines derived from traditional pharmacopoeia in member countries of the African Intellectual Property Organization (OAPI, 2003), two definitions have been proposed.

The first defines the pharmacopoeia, irrespective of its origin, as a collection or book containing monographs of medicinal plants, mineral or animal substances with physico-chemical and therapeutic properties identified and recognized by experts appointed by the competent authority.

It should be noted in passing, however, that the reference system is an official reference document for a country (national pharmacopoeia) or a group of countries (international, regional or sub-regional pharmacopoeia), with no legal status.

The second proposal highlights its African origins and defines traditional African pharmacopoeia as a body of knowledge, practices, preparation techniques and uses of plant, animal and/or mineral substances, used to diagnose, prevent and/or eliminate a physical, mental or social imbalance.

It's part of Africa's cultural heritage. Nowadays, it is transmitted orally or in written form from generation to generation.

The nuance between the two concepts lies in the fact that the practitioner of traditional medicine administers treatments with traditional remedies, unlike the pharmacopoeia specialist who limits himself to proposing, for therapeutic purposes, knowledge, practices and techniques for the preparation and use of endogenous substances (plant, animal and/or mineral), without taking upon himself the responsibility of administering care to the sick.

Traditional African Pharmacopoeia offers solutions to a wide range of illnesses, notably those whose biological origin has not been proven, and those whose microbial, bacteriological or viral origin has been established in a laboratory.

Pierre VERGER and Ming Anthony have published many of the results of their research into Traditional Medicine. These include

- "Issoyé : Médications de la mémoire chez les Yoruba en Afrique et au Brésil " ; médicaments et aliments, approche Ethnopharmacologique, Paris, Orstom, p. 174- 177 (Cf.1993- Compte -rendu du 2nd Colloquium on Ethnopharmacology) (ESE) Heidelberg, 24- 25 Mars p.49 ;
- In 1996, the team presented one of the causes of smallpox and its remedies in Yoruba tradition: "Sanponna god of smallpox and its remedies in Yoruba tradition" (in) healing, yesterday, today and tomorrow?

(1st international conference of anthropology and history of health and decease. 3rd European Colloquium on Ethnopharmacology, Genoa, Italy, May 29 to June 2, 1996). European Society of Ethnopharmacology, Erga Multimedia.

This work, which was the starting point for research into African medicinal plants, raised both hopes and questions among communities, including the colonial authorities. The colonial administration, which had scorned traditional recipes despite their often positive results, began to tolerate the coexistence of traditional and conventional medicine.

In the same spirit, as early as 1968, a scientific and technical committee of the Organization of African Unity (OAU) based in Lagos, Nigeria, published volumes 1 and 2 entitled "African Pharmacopoeia" in 1985 and 1988 respectively.

However, to be more socially useful and economically efficient, all these therapeutic potentialities need to be improved with a view to their integration into the national healthcare system.

In other circumstances, these words take the place of plant, animal or mineral preparations. In Traditional Medicine, they are called "active words" and are said to possess power.

### 2- The power of the word in Traditional Medicine

#### a) The power of the active word in Yoruba anthropology

In his book Ewé : Le verbe et le pouvoir des plantes chez les Yoruba (Nigeria-Benin), Pierre Fatumbi VERGER delves into Yoruba cultural anthropology to explain the power of the incantations that accompany the preparation of traditional therapeutic remedies.

"In traditional African culture, knowing the name of a person or thing means having some degree of control over it" (Robin Horton, 1967) quoted by Pierre Fatumbi VERGER).

- In 1976, in a paper entitled "The use of plants in Yoruba Traditional Medicine and its linguistic approach", in seminar series, (1976- 1977) 1$^{ère}$ partie, department of African language and literatures, of Ifè, p-242-295; Pierre VERGER addressed an important aspect of traditional medicine: the power of the spoken word. The author tried to demonstrate the importance of the word in traditional medicine.

During our fieldwork, we were concerned with the importance of the word (incantations) in traditional medicine.

We also sought to understand whether the verb acts before or during the preparation of the drug, or during its use.

The vast majority of over 95% of traditional practitioners we met on all our research sites affirmed that the spoken word has an important influence on the plant's efficacy. The spoken word has a long-term effect.

In some cases, it is advisable to pronounce the incantatory words throughout the treatment process, sometimes at the moment when the plant organ needed to prepare the remedy is removed. Through this ritual, the traditional practitioner uses powerful words to magnify the virtues of the plants. He urges them into action. Incantations can be used from the moment the plants are harvested, through to the preparation of the remedy and its use.

During treatment and each time the remedy is used, the patient or the treating traditional practitioner implores the plant's virtues to be more effective and, above all, faster in its healing actions.

#### b) The magnificence of the plant in Yoruba-Nago anthropology

"Every plant has a name that magnifies it and drives it to produce all its offensive effects on disease (particularly in its prevention or cure)" VERGER P. (1997).

In order to act and have an effect, words must be pronounced correctly. These are short sentences in which, very often, the verb indicates the expected action. The verb "to act" is one of the syllables in the name of the plant or ingredient used.

Speech is an integral part of traditional therapeutic knowledge and skills. Every learner must make it his or her own when transmitting it. Hence the ethnic character of African pharmacopoeia.

By way of illustration, Pierre VERGER mentions a remedy for coughs, classified on the divinatory tray (called odu obara ofun). Crush the leaves of quassia undulata (simaroubaceae) in the Yoruba national language oja, and mix with lemon juice (Citrus aurantifolia, rutaceae) in the Yoruba national language osin-oro -nbo or osin wèrè. Say the following before drinking three (03) tablespoons of the solution every morning:

Ója ja iko kuró l'orun mi

Óró-nbó bó iko kuró l'orun mi.

Which means:

Quassia undulata (Ója), breaks (ja) the cough (iko) in my throat.

Citrus aurantifolia (Óró-nbó) or lemon (in French), removes (bó) the cough I have in my throat (VERGER P.F. 1977).

The theoretical framework of this study would be incomplete without a brief presentation of the evolution of traditional medicine in Benin, Africa and the rest of the world.

## B- Evolution of Traditional Medicine

It's about the evolution of Traditional Medicine in the world, in Africa and in Benin.

### 1- In the world

In 1978, under the leadership of WHO and the United Nations Children's Fund (UNICEF), 134 health ministers from around the world signed the Alma Ata Declaration in Russia.

A new health strategy was adopted: Primary Health Care (PHC), with the objective of "health for all by the year 2000". The failure of previous prevention and mass-medicine policies was the driving force behind this new strategy.

The fundamental characteristics of these old policies were the continuing high prevalence of major endemic diseases, high infant mortality and low efficiency of overly expensive hospital medicine. For the first time, traditional medicine is recognized as an alternative, and traditional practitioners have become important partners in health care.

In addition, the World Health Organization has pointed out that, despite the abundance of allopathic treatments and techniques for chronic diseases, some patients do not find satisfactory solutions. These treatments and technologies have not been sufficiently effective, or have had negative effects.

In this regard, a recent study found that 78% of patients living with HIV/AIDS in the United States use some form of complementary or alternative medicine (Mason F.1995 Anderson W. et al 1993; and Ostrow M.J et al1997).

Another worldwide study identified only 193 negative events following acupuncture (including relatively minor events such as haematomas and dizziness) over a 15-year period (Studdert. D.M et al, 1998).

Complementary or alternative medicine (CAM) is considered more as a "complement" to allopathy than as an "alternative" to it (Astin J.A., 1998).

In 1998, the World Health Assembly reaffirmed its commitment to universal access to health care, calling on member states to provide the essential elements of primary health care (WHO, 15ème World Health Assembly, 1998).

As part of this requirement, and to improve access to essential medicines and encourage the role of Traditional Medicine in health systems, resolutions on the local production of traditional medicines, research and development of pharmacopoeia, the drafting of legislation specific to the practice of Traditional Medicine, and monographs on medicinal plants have been developed by the WHO and countries in the Afro region.

Since 1991, WHO has been developing guidelines and publishing technical and scientific guides to support research into Traditional Medicine. It also provides financial support to African countries for research into the safety and efficacy of Traditional Medicine therapies.

In its resolution "Promoting the role of traditional medicine in health systems", the WHO reaffirms the importance and potential of traditional medicine, and recommends the accelerated development of local production of so-called "traditional" medicines.

To achieve this, we need to help governments create an enabling environment, put in place guidelines for the formulation and evaluation of national policies in this field, and improve the economic and regulatory environment for local drug production.

In fact, the proven medical value and economic potential of medicinal plants when used judiciously means :

- investment in the development of human resources and research in Traditional Medicine;
- the mobilization of available resources for the development of Traditional Medicine health systems and their generalization throughout all health systems in Africa.

A brief presentation of the health situation in Africa will help us to better understand the strengths and weaknesses of the health system in our countries.

**2- In Africa**

In Africa, the actions of the Organization of African Unity (OAU) have been decisive in revaluing traditional medicine.

The Scientific, Technical and Research Commission of the OAU (STRC/OAU), the late father of the African Union (AU), has always considered the development of traditional medicine as one of its main activities. It has therefore set up an intra-African regional committee of experts to advise on this issue.

In 1985, she published the first volume of African Pharmacopoeia, followed by a second the same year.

Two centers of excellence have been identified, enabling scientific investigations to be carried out on African medicinal plant extracts. These are Obafèmi AWOLOWO University in Ile-Ifè, Nigeria, and the Mampong-Akwapim Medicinal Plant Research Center in Ghana.

At their July 2001 summit in Lusaka, Zambia, the Heads of State and Government of the African Union proclaimed the Decade of African Traditional Medicine for the period 20012010. The action plan put in place, as well as the mechanism for monitoring and reporting on the decade's plan, was presented and adopted in April 2003 at the first conference of African Union health ministers in Tripoli, Libya.

In addition, August 31 of each year has been declared African Traditional Medicine Day. A general framework guides member states in the formulation of their national strategies.

Eleven (11) priority areas have been identified, covering awareness-raising, legislation, institutional arrangements, information, education and communication, resource mobilization, training, cultivation and conservation of medicinal plants, protection of traditional medical knowledge, production of standardized African traditional medicines in quality and commercial quantities, partnerships, and evaluation, monitoring and reporting ( PETIT Pascale, 2007).

The U.A. summit held in Abuja, Nigeria, from January 24 to 31, 2005, reiterated the importance of research into traditional medicine, particularly with regard to the treatment of HIV/AIDS, tuberculosis, malaria and other infectious diseases.

To support the WHO's efforts in the field of primary healthcare, the African Union recommends that African countries strengthen their capacity to produce traditional medicines. This requires that Africans protect and preserve their cultural heritage and indigenous knowledge systems.

Finally, in April 2007, the 3$^{ème}$ ordinary session of the African Union Conference of Ministers of Health examined mid-term progress in implementing the decade's action plan.

Resolutions and declarations by international organizations in favor of traditional medicine and its integration into national healthcare systems have been instrumental in the adoption of policies to integrate traditional medicine into official healthcare systems in several countries, notably Benin.

### 3- In Benin

In Benin, we can distinguish three periods in the evolution of Traditional Medicine.

#### a) Colonial period

Until Benin gained independence, the only recognized and authorized health care methods were those of conventional medicine.

In 1965, five years after the country's accession to international sovereignty, the government of Dahomey (now Benin) timidly took the first step towards recognizing and promoting Traditional Medicine.

By decree no. 1146/ MSP/ DGM / DRMPT of March 26 1965, the Department of Research into Traditional Medicine and Pharmacopoeia was created and placed under the supervision of the Ministry of Public Health.

#### b) Revolutionary period

This era was marked by the fight against obscurantism, witchcraft and fetishism. Revolutionary power fought everything that embodied tradition. For revolutionaries, traditional power was an obstacle to development. According to them, traditional practices prevented the rain from falling.

For an agriculture based on rainfall, the absence of rain is the first obstacle to agricultural production.

It was a time of confusion between cultural values and traditions. Benin had lost much of its cultural heritage.

Paradoxically, at the same time, the importance of traditional medicine was recognized and promoted by the revolutionary authorities, who quickly realized that the country's financial resources would not allow them to offer people equitable access to mass healthcare.

On November 30, 1972, President Mathieu KEREKOU announced his government's commitment to recognizing and revaluing traditional medicine with the following declaration: "Combining modern and traditional medicine for the well-being of our masses and the progress of medical practice in Dahomey, recognizing the importance of our pharmacopoeia" (Program Speech, 1972).

This declaration marks the beginning of a new era for Traditional Medicine in the country. It emerged from the clandestinity into which it had been forced by colonial rule. And the number of self-declared traditional practitioners and practitioner associations immediately increased.

Happy intentions to associate Traditional Medicine with official health care have been realized. A framework for collaboration between the two types of medicine was implemented. But the experiment soon showed its limitations.

The climate of trust that should characterize this collaboration very quickly turned sour, and was transformed into a climate of mistrust and hostility between the players.

Traditional practitioners work under the orders and control of their colleagues in modern medicine, who boast a superiority complex conferred on them by their standardized diploma training.

Almost all of the experimental centers for collaboration between traditional and modern medicine have ceased to operate, due to a lack of trust between the players and, above all, a lack of motivation for the traditional practitioners working in this unusual setting.

Traditional healers' services are not fully appreciated. They rightly or wrongly equate certain behaviors of health workers with a lack of consideration for their art and for themselves.

Furthermore, in 1979, in view of the environment characterized by a leadership war between the actors grouped within the antagonistic associations in which traditional medicine was practiced, the Marxist government dissolved all these associations of traditional medicine practitioners. Selection criteria for traditional practitioners were defined.

In 1986, the decree recognizing the status of the National Association of Traditional Medicine Practitioners of Benin (ANAPRAMETRAB) was issued. This national association is unique and aims to improve the contribution of traditional practitioners to health promotion, in close collaboration with the Ministry of Health.

In 1996, the Ministry of Health created the National Pharmacopoeia and Traditional Medicine Program (PNPMT). For the time being, this program remains the reference structure for implementing the government's policy of promoting and upgrading traditional medicine in Benin.

We can't talk about traditional medicine without considering its raw materials.

Plants are the main resources of traditional medicine, and natural flora is the main source of plant material.

For this reason, it will be useful and timely to specify in the study how Benin's flora is managed.

### c) Managing Benin's flora

Article 1 of law no. 93-009 of July 02 1993 on the forest regime in the Republic of Benin[er] , sets out the framework for the management, protection and exploitation of natural flora in Benin.

Article 2 of the implementing decree (decree no. 96- 271 of July 02, 1996), which sets out the application of the law of July 02, 1993, defines forests in Benin.

Under the terms of this article, forests are defined as land with a vegetation cover, including mangroves, with the exception of agricultural crops which may :

- To supply wood or non-agricultural products;
- Shelter wildlife and other biological resources;
- Beneficial effects on the soil, climate, biodiversity, water regime or natural environment; or
- fulfil recreational, cultural and scientific functions.

In Africa in general, and in Benin in particular, especially in rural areas, natural flora is still the basic pharmacy for people who can't afford the cost of conventional medicine.

Despite all the protection and regulatory measures in place, Benin's forests are still exposed to serious natural pressures and threats as a result of man's actions on nature.

These threats and pressures are called :

- Overexploitation of plant resources, with the main activities being the harvesting of firewood, abusive exploitation of timber and the felling of shrubs for charcoal;
- Illegal bushfires;
- The use of cultivation methods such as shifting cultivation and mechanized farming;
- Climate change;
- The systematic destruction of certain plant species through ignorance or misunderstanding.

In recent years, Benin has experienced strong demographic pressure. This predominantly poor population uses fossil fuels for their domestic needs, putting heavy pressure on the country's flora.

A lucrative business is developing around firewood. Urban centers are supplied daily from rural areas.

In addition to this trade in firewood, Benin's flora is exploited for other commercial purposes.

On a national and international level, the timber market has become as flourishing as mining resources. This market has become a major economic issue, with the gradual development of Benin's timber industry as a result.

Among other pressures, every year Benin's flora falls victim to illegal bush fires and traditional cultivation practices such as slash-and-burn agriculture.

In addition, Benin's natural flora is under pressure from poor methods of harvesting plants for use in traditional medicine.

Finally, climate change is also a major threat to Benin's flora, as is the mechanization of agriculture.

These few images from the field illustrate the extent of the pressures and threats facing Benin's flora.

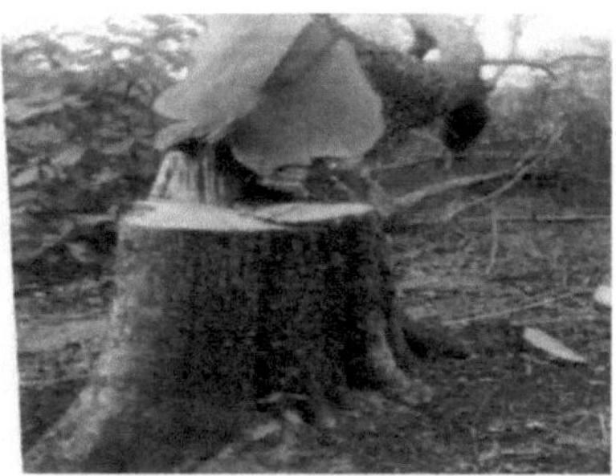

**Photo 1:** CONOCARPUS leïocarpus, a virtuous plant called Agni in the local SABÈ language, felled for processing into logs.

The plant has anti-measles properties when combined with the CAJANUS CAJAN plant, called OTILI in the local SABÈ language. The decoction is used in a warm bath and as a drink three times a day (morning, noon and evening).

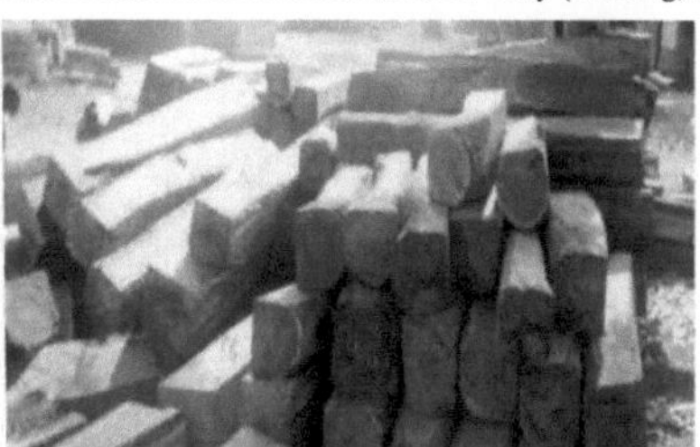

**Photo 2**: A log dump at Kaboua in the commune of Savè.
(**Photo: Tiamiou AKPONNE, December 2009**).

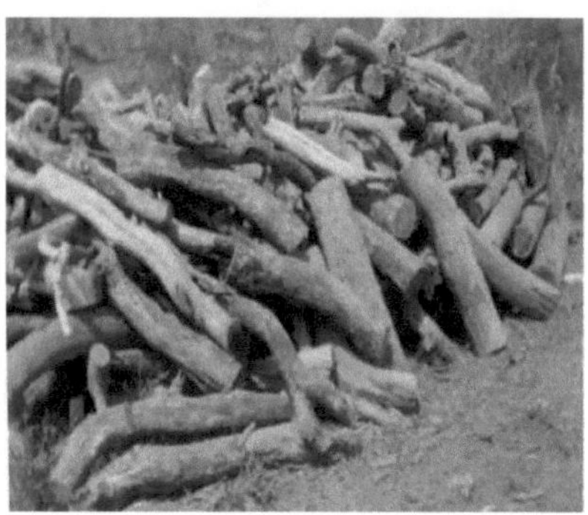

**Photo 3**: One of the many fuelwood markets in Alafia, Kaboua district (**Photo: Tiamiou AKPONNE, December 2009**).

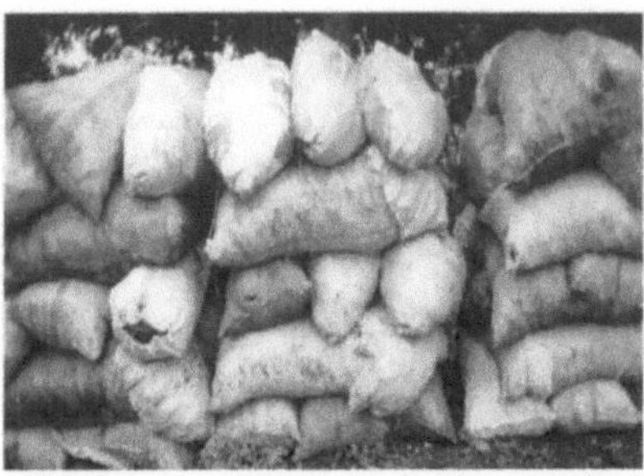

**Photo 4:** A partial view of a charcoal sack warehouse in Chayagbangba, Kaboua district **(Photo: Tiamiou AKPONNE, December 2009).**

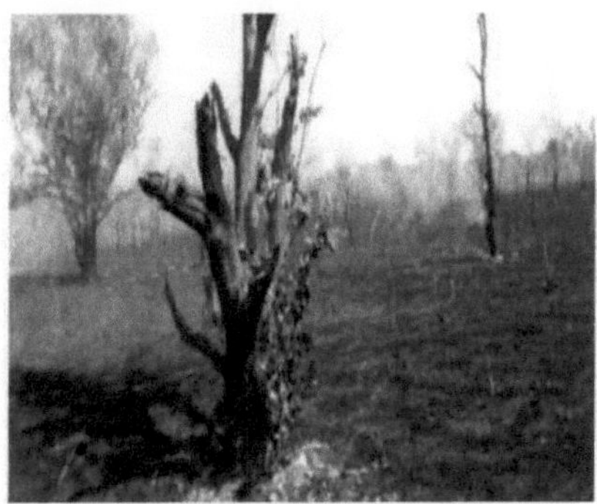

Photo 5: A cashew plantation decimated by illegal bushfire (Photo: Tiamiou AKPONNE, December 2009)

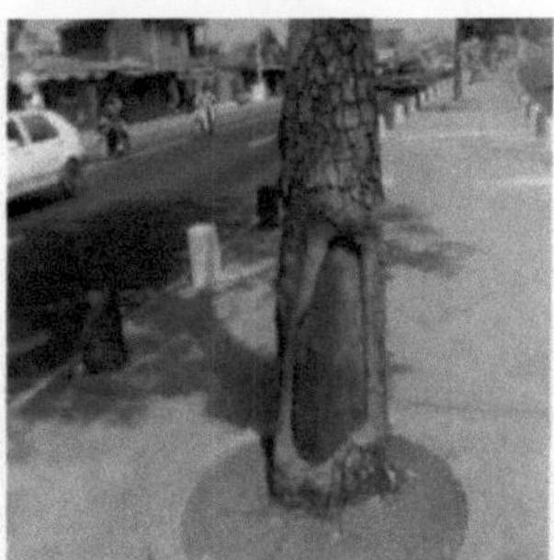

**Photo 6:** Poor bark removal is detrimental to plant survival
(**Photo: Tiamiou AKPONNE, December, 2009**)

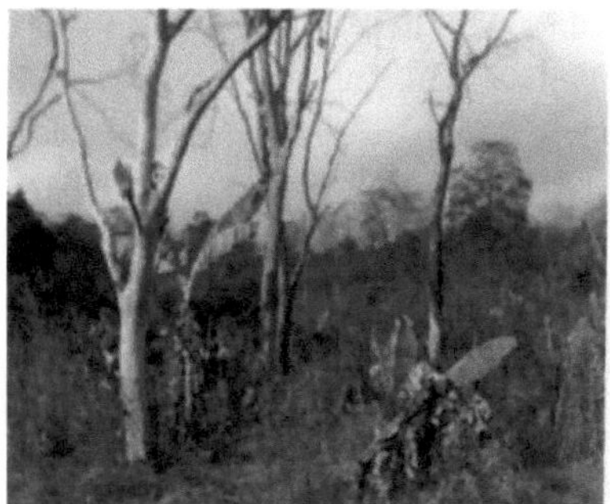

**Photo 7:** The fallow technique of abandoning a field to the mercy of bush fires after several years is also harmful to plants.

**(Photo: Tiamiou AKPONNE, December 2009)**

The combination of these phenomena dangerously jeopardizes the sustainability of plant resources for traditional medicine in Benin. Hence the need to make the generalization of botanical gardens a priority in the national policy for integrating traditional medicine into the Beninese health system.

Finally, to conclude the study on the evolution of traditional medicine in Benin, it is also important to address the legal framework governing the practice of this medicine.

### d) Legal framework for the practice of Traditional Medicine.

Since independence, the Beninese legislator, who succeeded the colonial legislator, has not yet considered legislation on the development of Traditional Medicine and Pharmacopoeia.

However, some regulatory provisions relating to the conditions of practice of Traditional Medicine and the recognition of the national association of Traditional Medicine practitioners are set out in the association's statutes and internal regulations (ANAPRAMETRAB).

There is also another decree laying down the conditions for the practice of Traditional Medicine in Benin, not forgetting the inter-ministerial order laying down the rules for advertising Traditional Medicine and Pharmacopoeia.

Together, these regulatory texts constitute the only legal arsenal for traditional medicine and pharmacopoeia in Benin.

By decree no. 86- 69 of March 3, 1986 laying down the statutes and internal regulations of the national association of traditional medicine practitioners in Benin, the government recognized the national association of traditional medicine practitioners in Benin.

However, this recognition alone was not enough to organize this informal sector. It was not until 2001 that decree n° 2001- 036 of February 15, 2001 laid down the principles of professional ethics and the conditions for the practice of traditional medicine in the Republic of Benin.

To put an end to the informal market in Traditional Pharmacopoeia medicines and to the illegal practice of Traditional Medicine, the Minister of Health and the Minister of Communication and Promotion of New Technologies, by interministerial decree no. 9969 / MSP/DC.SGM/DPED/C-P/MT/SA of November 03, 2004, regulating advertising of Traditional Pharmacopoeia and Medicine in Benin, set the conditions for advertising in this field.

In accordance with the provisions of article 3 of the aforementioned decree, traditional medicines that have been registered with the pharmacopoeia directorate and whose therapeutic efficacy has been certified by the laboratory authorized to carry out the clinical test are authorized to be advertised.

Before the advertisement is published, article 4 of the same decree requires the press organization concerned to ensure that the words "vu bon à publier" (in view of publication), signed by the person in charge of the pharmacopoeia, are entered on the order form.

Registration is subject to one condition: to be registered, traditional medicines must come from authors who have themselves been registered with the structure in charge of pharmacopoeia and traditional medicine.

Notwithstanding the provisions of article 11 of this decree, which punishes any breach of the regulations with a penalty and a fine ranging from 100,000 to 500,000 F CFA, offers of medicines from the pharmacopoeia and traditional healthcare continue to appear with impunity on radio and television stations and in newspaper columns.

In a letter dated April 11, 2007, the Minister of Health reminded media managers of the regulations governing advertising of pharmacopoeia and traditional medicine in Benin.

Advertising through the media is still the only channel best suited to health service providers in traditional medicine, especially in urban areas.

Anyone can stand up without any formalities and proclaim themselves a tradipratician, offering traditional health care or traditional medicines to the population. "This practice, which is contrary to the regulations in force in Benin, leads to uncontrolled consumption of these products, with health, economic and social consequences that are still difficult to assess" (Ms, 2007).

At the Direction des pharmacies et du médicament, the body responsible for receiving applications for registration, we were told that applications for registration of traditional pharmacopoeia medicines are still pending for lack of an appropriate legal framework.

According to those in charge of the legal department of the Pharmacy and Medicines Directorate, the texts are currently being drafted.

To compensate for the inadequacy or absence of regulations governing the production of traditional medicines, the African Intellectual Property Organization (OAPI), under the impetus of the World Health Organization (WHO), has initiated a reference system for the harmonization of approval procedures for medicines derived from traditional pharmacopoeia, for the benefit of its sixteen (16) member states.

As Benin is a member of this organization, it is in the interests of its policy of promoting Traditional Medicine and Pharmacopoeia to bring the provisions of the referential into line with its draft law on Traditional Pharmacopoeia and Medicine, which has been in the pipeline since 2008, according to information gathered from officials at the National Traditional Pharmacopoeia and Medicine Program.

OAPI's initiative to promote medicines from traditional pharmacopoeia is, and will remain, a welcome step in the policy of integrating traditional medicine into the healthcare systems of OAPI member countries.

Medicines derived from traditional pharmacopoeia are based on traditional therapeutic knowledge. The therapeutic virtues of medicinal plants have been mastered by traditional health practitioners since the dawn of time.

## C- Benin's health system

The health system encompasses all the material, human, financial and organizational resources deployed by the State or its branches to provide health care for the population.

### 1- Sanitary coverage

### a) Organization of the health system in Benin

**Table 1**: Organization of the health system in Benin

| LEVELS | STRCTURES | HOSPITAL AND SOCIAL-HEALTH INSTITUTIONS | SPECIALTIES |
|---|---|---|---|

| CENTRAL OR NATIONAL<br><br><br><br>INTERMEDIARE Or DEPARTEMENTAL<br><br><br>PERIPHERAL OR COMMUNAL | Ministry of Health (MS)<br><br><br>Management Departmental Health (DDS)<br><br><br>Sanitary zone (Zone Office) | -National Hospital and University Center (CNHU- HKM)<br><br>Center Hospitalier Départemental (CHD)<br><br><br>- Zone Hospital (HZ)<br>- Community Health Center (CSC)<br>- Center d'Action de la Solidarité et d'Evolution de la Santé (CASES) - Private health training courses<br>-District Health Center (CSA)<br>- Maternity wards and Dispensaries<br><br>- Village Health Unit (UVS) | - Medicine - Pediatrics<br>- Surgery - Gynaecology<br>- Obstetrics - Radiology - Laboratory - ENT Ophthalmology Other specialties<br>- Medicine - Pediatrics<br>- Surgery - Gyneco-obstetrics - Radiology<br>- Laboratory - ENT Ophthalmology<br>- Other specialties<br><br>- General Medicine<br>- Emergency surgery<br>- Gyneco-obstetrics - Dispensary<br>- Maternity ward<br>- Literacy<br>- Leisure<br>- Radiology<br>- Laboratory<br>- Pharmacy -Dispensary<br>- Maternity -Pharmacy or pharmacy depot -Care<br>- Births - Pharmacy case |
|---|---|---|---|

Source: Yearbook of Health Statistics 2002 (MS)

Benin's healthcare system is characterized by a number of structural and management shortcomings. The structure is based on the administrative division of the country. The health system in Benin is administered at central level by the Ministry of Health (MOH), at departmental or intermediate level by the Departmental Health Directorate (DDS), and at peripheral or communal level by the Zone Hospitals (HZ).

At district level, the district health centers act as the public health administration.

The inconsistencies of such an organization are as follows:

- private health facilities are not under the control of the health administration
- unbalanced distribution of sanitary facilities
- the distance of certain health centers from urban areas
- poor or non-functioning health centers in certain localities.

**b) Health system management in Benin**

The health system encompasses human, financial and material resources.

There have been a number of difficulties in the training policy for resources. The suspension of training for several years at the national medico-social institute (INMES) is an illustration of the planning difficulties.

Every year, the country's two universities deliver dozens of doctors to the job market, and the system struggles to keep them fully occupied.

## 2- Epidemiological status

**The aim here is to answer the following question:**

What are the people of Benin suffering from?

### a) Common ailments

Based on the statistics of the health system in Benin, the most common diseases encountered are :

- malaria;
- acute respiratory infections;
- gastrointestinal disorders;
- trauma;
- Diarrhea;
- anemias ;
- HIV/AIDS;
- dermatological conditions;
- hypertension;
- urogenital disorders;
- osteoarticular and some other conditions.

It should be pointed out here that the study essentially focused on cases of illness known to the health facilities.

This clarification is all the more necessary as some diseases are beyond the reach of modern medicine. Hepatitis B and C, for example, are not supernatural diseases.

These illnesses are of a supranatural nature (many cases of bewitchment, witchcraft or bad luck) and their effective treatment is sometimes beyond the competence of health facilities.

As a result, there are many pathologies that cannot be effectively managed by traditional healthcare methods.

### b) Benin's healthcare system

Benin's healthcare system is heterogeneous, combining a public and a private sector.

> **Public sector**

As part of the implementation of the primary healthcare strategy, the organizational chart of healthcare structures is as follows:

- A national reference hospital in Cotonou. This is the Centre National Hospitalier Universitaire Hubert Koutoukou MAGA (CNHU/HKM).
- Five (05) Centres Hospitaliers Départementaux(CHD) located in the country's six departmental capitals, with the exception of Cotonou, which already houses the national university hospital center.

  Each departmental center now covers two departments, in line with the new territorial division:

  - Center hospitalier départemental Ouémé-Plateau (CHD/Ouémé-Plateau) ;
  - Center hospitalier départemental Mono-Kouffo (CHD/ Mono -Kouffo) ;
  - Center hospitalier départemental Zou- Collines (CHD/Zou- Collines) ;
  - Center hospitalier départemental Borgou-Alibori (CHD/ Borgou- Alibori) ;
  - Center hospitalier départemental Atacora- Donga (CHD/Atacora- Donga).

Each of the country's seventy-seven (77) communes has a health center known as a Centre Communal de Sant2 (CCS). These communal health centers are grouped into Health Zones, headed by a Zone Hospital (HZ), which is the local referral center.

Village health units (UVS) are set up in villages with a high concentration of people.

- **Private sector**

The freeze on recruitment of graduates from medical schools and faculties has encouraged the establishment of many medical practices. But for some time now, religious denominations have been making their presence felt in the health sector in the form of non-governmental organizations. Large faith-based health centers offer a wide range of healthcare services to fill the gap created by the public sector.

### 3- Drug supply in Benin

Medicines are supplied by both the public and private sectors.

The public sector is covered by the central purchasing office for essential medicines and medical consumables (CAME). The national laboratory for quality control of essential medicines and medical consumables carries out chemical analysis of medicines before they are authorized for marketing.

The private sector is managed by private operators who import, produce and distribute medicines.

Here, too, non-governmental organizations and other religious bodies receive donations of medicines which, unfortunately, escape the regulatory provisions in force. There is therefore an informal sector of drug imports in Benin that is hard to pin down. The parallel drug market remains a challenge for the official health system in Africa in general, and in Benin in particular.

### 4- Training

Three levels characterize the training of health workers in Benin:

- The lower level trains health nurses.

  This training was provided by the Ecole Nationale des Infirmiers Assistants du Bénin, which recruited nurses with a primary school certificate (CEP). But for some time now, this training has been interrupted;

- The intermediate level is that of state-qualified nurses (IDE) trained at the Institut National Médico- Social (INMES), a public technical and vocational training establishment.

Access to the entrance examination for this school is now subject to the Baccalauréat rather than the BEPC, as was previously the case. The higher level trains doctors capable of carrying out care, prevention and health education tasks, as well as specialists in general surgery, gynecology-obstetrics, internal medicine, pediatrics and psychiatry.

Training is provided in the faculties and schools of Benin's two universities:

- University of Abomey - Calavi (FSS/UAC);
- and the University of Parakou (FM/UP).

### 5- Human resources

The development of the health sector relies on the services of a large workforce. The health personnel used by the Ministry include doctors, nurses, midwives, laboratory technicians and radiology technicians. Health workers also provide services in the private sector.

However, public health facilities are still suffering from staff shortages. The departments of Donga, Atacora, Alibori, Collines, Couffo and Plateau have 20,000 inhabitants per doctor.

### 6- Health financing in Benin

Health financing remains one of the biggest challenges facing the healthcare system.

According to statistical data from the Ministry of Health's Department of Studies and Planning, the evolution of the health sector budget from 2007 to 2010 is as follows in thousands of FCFA :

- 2007 = 64,881 or 7.98% of the general government budget ;

- 2008 = 73,921 or 7.23% of the general State budget ;
- 2009 = 111,415 or 8.99% of the general State budget;

 2010 = 82,462 or 6.12% of the State's general budget.

Community participation through community financing, a corollary of the Bamako initiative, is an essential element in the smooth running of Benin's healthcare system. It is managed by the commune management committee (COGEC) and the arrondissement management committee (COGEA).

These different structures promote and develop community participation in health activities;

The contribution of our partners to health development in Benin is not negligible.

Benin's health development partners include :

- Islamic Development Bank (IDB);
- Fonds d'Aide à la Coopération (FAC);
- Development Aid Fund(FAD) ;
- United Nations Population Fund (UNFPA) ;
- World Health Organization (WHO);
- Japan;
- Switzerland;
- USA;
- UNAIDS ;
- The Federal Republic of Germany
- Belgium
- United Nations Development Programme
- Kuwait Fund for Development.

To achieve the objective assigned to the study, the research was based on a methodology that favored the documentary approach and the field as the main sources of information.

# CHAPTER 2: METHODOLOGICAL APPROACH

## A- Research stages

Documentary research was carried out in documentation centers and in the field.

### 1- Documentation centers

The documentation and information center of the United Nations system, the archives of the Center for Research and Experimentation in Traditional Medicine (CREMPT) in Porto-Novo, and the computer library of the School of African Heritage (EPA) in the same city, all played a major role in the summary of documentary information sources.

#### a) Training seminars and workshops

The reports of the seminars and workshops in which we took part as speakers also made a significant contribution to the documentary orientation of the research.

The first workshop, held at the Institut de Développement et des Echanges Endogènes (IDEE) in Ouidah from July 16 to 18, 2008, organized by the Programme National de la Pharmacopée et de la Médecine Traditionnelle (PNPMT), focused on the validation of a clinical research protocol for the evaluation of remedies used in traditional medicine to treat HIV/AIDS in Benin.

This seminar marks an important step in the Benin government's commitment to promoting traditional medicine as a means of finding endogenous solutions to the fight against HIV/AIDS, which today represents a major development challenge for the black continent, where the disease claims the most victims.

The second workshop is a follow-up to the Ouidah workshop. It took place in Bohicon from August 28 to 29, 2008, and focused on a consultation meeting with national traditional medicine players involved in the evaluation of remedies used in traditional medicine for the treatment of HIV/AIDS. The purpose of the meeting was to present the protocol to traditional medicine practitioners.

### 2- Development of field survey tools

This exercise first enabled us to better circumscribe the study problem and then led to the development of data collection tools used in the field as part of the surveys.

In addition, research has provided indications that characterize traditional medicine in its foundations, approaches and practice.

For the practitioner of traditional medicine, the concept of illness is different from that of the agent of conventional medicine.

The traditional belief is that illness can be caused by a number of factors. These factors can be divided into natural and unnatural causes (Felharber et al, 1997).

Natural causes of illness include germs, age-related diseases and accidents.

An object or matter (living or non-living, visible or invisible) can enter the body through the mouth (eating it), the skin, the nostril (sniffing or breathing it in) or through evil spirits. Also, anything (object or organism) can enter the body through walking (barefoot or wearing shoes). Once inside the body, it can migrate or settle in a particular organ, causing it to become diseased.

Unnatural causes of disease include witchcraft and spirits. These abnormal causes have not been scientifically exploited or proven. Witchcraft refers to the activity of a few individuals who cause harm or illness through misuse of their natural abilities or knowledge of medicines used for the purpose of not curing. Spirits refer to individuals who have died in unfortunate events or accidents, and who have not been properly buried. These spirits haunt individuals who are not related to them. Induced bad actions can take many forms: violent actions, madness, etc.

In conclusion, documentary research is a decisive stage in the preparation of a field survey. For the purposes of the methodology, the presentation of the research sector and the justification of the choice have not escaped the present study.

**B- Field research**

**1- Presentation and justification of the research framework**

**a) Location of study areas**

- Kinta district in the Agbangnizoun district on the Abomey plateau;
- The arrondissement of Kétou - Centre in the Commune of Kétou on the Ouémé plateau in south-east Benin;
- Kaboua district in the Savè commune in central France;
- Nikki- Centre district in the northern commune of Nikki - Eastern Benin.

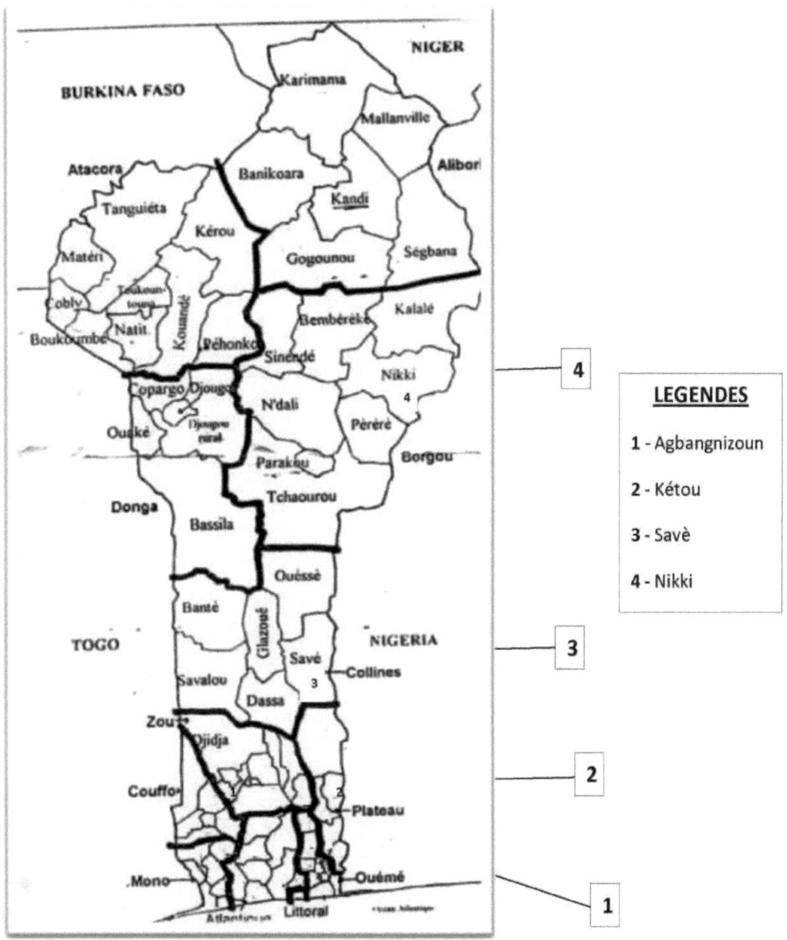

**Source:** INSAE, 2002 (adapted to our study sectors by ourselves)

## b) Presentation and rationale for choice of study areas

As it was impossible to carry out the survey across the whole country, we limited ourselves to four (04) localities in Benin. The four localities were chosen on the basis of socio-cultural differences and belonging to well-defined agro-ecological and geographical zones.

These are the arrondissement of Kinta in the commune of Agbangnizoun in south-east Benin, the arrondissement of Kétou-Centre in the commune of Kétou in the east of the country, the arrondissement of Kaboua in the commune of Savè in the center, and the arrondissement of Nikki-Centre in the commune of Nikki in north-east Benin.

> **Criteria linked to the history and continuity of our traditions.**

With its long history, Traditional Medicine is part of Africa's cultural heritage. It has never ceased to serve peoples and contribute to the health and socio-economic development of communities.

In the commune of Agbangnizoun, for example, pharmacopoeia is listed among the top local resources. The commune's development plan justifies its health, economic and social importance with the following statement: "Traditional medicine is the main recourse for the vast majority of the population.

The commune is recognized as an important center for pharmacopoeia in the southern part of our country. This activity supports a significant proportion of the Commune's population" (PDC Agbangnizoun 2004-2008).

In the Baatombou(Bariba) community of Nikki, people are still very attached to cultural and ancestral values. This is demonstrated by their allegiance to their King on the occasion of the Gaani festivities, a symbol of unity and respect for the traditions of the Wassagari peoples.

The Nagos of Kétou and Savè take great care to safeguard and perpetuate their cultural heritage (ASA) bequeathed to them by their common ancestor **ODUDUA**.

All these different national communities have appropriated traditional medicine and apply it on the basis of their social and cultural realities. Hence the name traditional medicine, i.e. medicine based on realities drawn from traditions.

The choice of localities where cultural and ancestral values are still safeguarded is the main motivation.

After consultation with our two thesis supervisors, the localities of the Abomey plateau, the Kétou, Savè and Nikki regions were identified as reference areas for the perpetuation of ancestral traditions.

In these societies, the brotherhood of hunters played and still plays an important role in the protection and defense of the kingdom and the health of the population.

Moreover, these regions are known for the peaceful cohabitation of the different communities that live there, even if in recent years a few hotbeds of tension have been ignited and quickly extinguished.

In all these communes, different ethnic groups live together in mutual respect for their cultural differences. This intermingling of communities is a positive element that justifies the country's cultural diversity.

> **Different study areas**

In the Agbangnizoun region, the land becomes increasingly fertile as you descend towards the Couffo river valley. The ferralitic soils associated with the vast sheets of ferruginous cuirasses of the Kétou plateau offer agricultural possibilities and allow the growth of a wide variety of flower species.

The Savè region, a climatic transition zone, is home to several types of vegetation and offers farming areas between the hollows of the massifs and along the banks of watercourses, the most important of which are the Ouémé and Okpara rivers.

In the Nikki region, the soils are more homogeneous. This gives greater agricultural potential, but the climate here is Sudanian.

From one region to another, differences in relief, climate, vegetation and hydrography are major determinants of soil composition and plant chemical elements.

For example, the OCINUM GRATISSINUM (mosquito plant, tea bush or fever leaf) grown in Kétou does not produce the same effects as that produced in Kinta in the commune of Agbangnizoun, for the simple reason that in the Kétou region, located on a low-lying plateau (between 100 and 200 m), impoverished, desaturated, ferralitic soils with indurations have developed, associated with vast aquifers bearing sparse vegetation.

The district of Kaboua in the commune of Savè, a crossroads region par excellence between the south and north of the country, has an agro-ecological advantage favorable to the cultivation of plant species from the north or south.

The difference between the soils of the four selected regions is also a comparative advantage in terms of the scope of our study. In the Agbangnizoun region, the soils are homogeneous: sandy-loamy, shallow and rapidly leaching, they are rapidly impoverished by intensive cultivation.

In the Kétou region, on the other hand, located on a low-lying plateau (between 100 and 200 m), impoverished soils with a low ferralitic content, desaturated and indurated, have developed, associated with vast blankets bearing little vegetation.

In the commune of Savè, the soils are underlain by the Precambrian basement of the crystalline peneplain, composed of granite, biotle gneiss and pegmatite veins. The bedrock is covered by sandy-clay formations of varying thickness, renowned for their permeability and low nitrogen and potassium content.

Soils in the Nikki commune are also tropical ferruginous. But these are soils of varying depths, with generally good permeability and porosity. They have mineral reserves, high acidity and low saturation.

These soils appear to be the result of deep, intense alteration of nutritive matter. Almost everywhere, they display a high degree of physical homogeneity. Highly cultivated, the soils are sensitive to erosion, with major constraints on farming.

Benin's flora varies from region to region. In the Agbangnizoun region, the plant cover is made up of shrubs with the presence of a few trees, dominated by the cultivated oil palm (ELAEIS GUINEENSIS).

There are also gallery forests and sacred forest islands along the rivers.

Kétou is dominated by wooded savannah, with a few forests such as the Kétou and Dogo classified forests and the Adakplamè sacred forest.

The flora of the Savè region consists of savannah dotted with trees and shrubs. There are still pockets of forest, including the 20,500-hectare Ouémé-Boukou classified forest, and gallery forests along the Ouémé River and other watercourses.

Nikki's flora is made up of wooded savannahs, trees and shrubs. Sparse forests are also present in places.

In the various zones, the most common species are :

- COMBRETUM nilgricans (Fon = koudékoudé or hégnimalé; and Bariba = koulogoutémini)
- DETARIUM microcarpum (Nago = iyédé ; Fon = dakpa ; Bariba = béhérou)
- GARDENIA eruberubescens (Nago = agni; Fon = koubo or dakpla; and Bariba igou or hirou)
- GARDENIA ternifolia (Nago = Kikiba; Bariba = Ganou)

The woody species found in fields and fallows are those spared from human pressure because of their socio-economic importance. These are essentially :

- VITELLARIA paradoxa
- PARKIA biglobosa (Nago = Ugba ; Fon = ahouatin ; Bariba = donm ; French Néré)

The woody recrus often found in fields and fallows are :

- DANIELLIA oliveri (Nago = iya or uya; Fon = za; Bariba = gnabou or gnabourou and in French = copalier africain de balsam).
- PARINARI curatellifolia (Nago = jaoké; Fon = kotama or houantou; Bariba = pakoukou or bawourou).

The floristic composition of the herbaceous stratum varies with the age of the formation. The dominant species are :

- PENNISETUM polystachion
- INDIGOFERA SPP
- TEPHROSIA pedicellata.

Given the field of study (Traditional Medicine), where almost all information is shrouded in secrecy, to reach the target populations we used information-gathering techniques that enabled us to achieve our objectives.

**2- Data collection**

**a) Collection techniques**

In the present study, data collection was based on direct contact with the populations concerned, interviews and group activities.

Also known as "participant observation", direct contact is based on scrutinizing local realities "from the inside", as close as possible to the people who live them, and in constant interaction with them.

The use of this tool, which turns the researcher into a witness, has enabled us to better understand the environment of traditional medicine in Benin.

During the course of the survey, we visited traditional practitioners in villages to observe at close quarters the therapeutic methods used to treat illnesses.

This method enabled us to put into perspective the information collected by declarative means. As a result, we were able to obtain data on traditional remedies used by traditional practitioners to treat certain illnesses, which was difficult to obtain by interview. It also enabled us to distinguish, albeit with difficulty, between traditional medicine and certain occult practices.

Finally, participant observation enabled us to appreciate the traditional therapeutic itinerary of the communities and to experience first-hand the management of illnesses by traditional practitioners.

In addition, interviews were conducted with the help of an interpreter where necessary, particularly among populations without schooling.

This technique has been used mainly with traditional practitioners, merchants of traditional medicine raw materials and certain neutral people (who don't belong to any other target group).

It provided important information on experiences, perceptions and opinions on the practice of Traditional Medicine.

For a proper understanding of social phenomena, it is necessary to account for representations. The notes and transcriptions from individual interviews with target persons, using an interview guide, formed the largest part of the corpus of data collected.

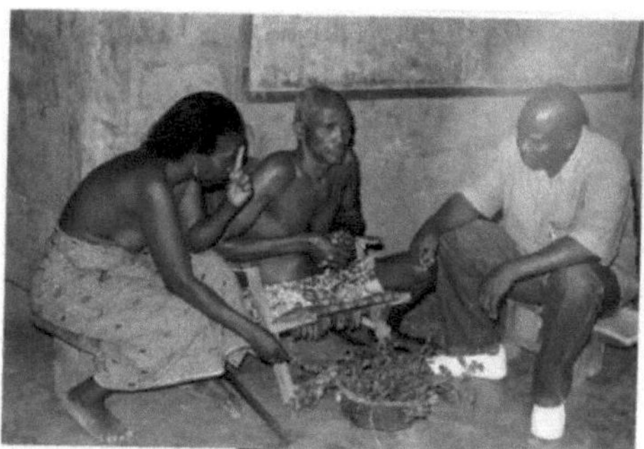

Photo 8: Interview with a Kinta traditional practitioner couple in the village of Danli (Photo: Claude MASSENON, March 2009).

For a better view of the populations surveyed, a breakdown by socio-professional category was carried out and is presented in the following tables:

**b) Breakdown of samples by socio-professional category**

A breakdown of our sample is shown in the following table:

**Table 2**: Target samples

| Order no. | Socioprofessional categories | Number of respondents |
| --- | --- | --- |
| 01 | Traditional healers | 84 |
| 02 | Merchants of Traditional Medicine Resources | 84 |
| 03 | Patients | 68 |
| 04 | Neutral people | 76 |
| 05 | Health agents | 84 |
| **Total** | **04 samples** | **396** |

In addition to interviews with each of the samples, we also held discussions. A total of eight (08) discussion sessions were held in all twelve (12) villages in the four (04) geographical areas of our study.

Two sessions were held in each arrondissement and commune. The following table shows the breakdown of the animated discussion sessions.

**Table 2**: Breakdown of moderated discussion sessions

| Communes | Boroughs | Villages | Number of interviews | Number of participants |
| --- | --- | --- | --- | --- |
| 01- Nikki | Nikki- center | Nikki<br>Kpariséro | 02 | 35 |
| 02- Savè | Kaboua | Kaboua, Okounfo, Alafia | 02 | 37 |
| 03- Kétou | Kétou center | Kétou<br>Odo-Mèta | 02 | 32 |
| 04 - Agbangnizoun | Kinta | Kinta, Danhi, Ahissatogon | 02 | 31 |
| **Total** | **04** | **12** | **08** | **135 people** |

In total, based on samples of traditional practitioners, patients, traders in traditional medicine raw materials, health workers and neutrals, the survey covered a population of six hundred and seventy-six (676) people.

Group activities were carried out on three samples:

- Traditional healers ;
- Patients ;
- Neutral people.

> **With traditional practitioners**

To carry out this activity, we relied on the local authorities, particularly the village chiefs. The meetings were held at the homes of the local presidents of the association of traditional medicine practitioners. Discussions focused on the organization and practice of traditional medicine in their locality, the difficulties encountered and progress made, and the outlook for the future.

> **With patients**

Encounters with patients who had chosen to be treated with traditional medicine had not been easy.

Indeed, in the communities, the disease is a taboo that is not often exposed in public. The decision to turn to a traditional practitioner is taken with great discretion.

Thanks to the understanding of the traditional healers and the cooperation of the health workers, we were able to obtain permission to see patients. Some of these patients were seen by their traditional healers, while others were seen at the health centers when traditional treatment had failed.

These meetings often take place in complete secrecy on busy days at the centers and at the residence of the center manager.

These group discussions helped to clarify information gathered individually during interviews on traditional medicine practices. They were organized in all four zones surveyed (with a total of two discussions per zone).

> **With neutral people**

The term "neutral" refers to people who are neither traditional healers, nor health workers, nor sick people. In other words, at the time of the survey, they were not being treated by a traditional practitioner, nor were they in need of treatment using traditional medicine.

Here too, the support of health facility managers was remarkable. We used the prenatal consultation channel to interview women, sometimes accompanied by their spouse or a family member. Using the interview guide, we were able to clarify a number of questions about traditional medicine.

The question of why these communities choose traditional medicine was not forgotten, and the various contributions shed light on the many points that will be important for the rest of the survey.

This methodological orientation, based on the use of a variety of data collection methods, generated information that enabled us to cover the full range of representations and categories.

The following table shows the breakdown of group events by location.

**Table 3**: Breakdown of Focus projects by location

| Communes | Boroughs | Villages | Number of focus groups | Number of participants |
|---|---|---|---|---|
| 01- Nikki | | Nikki<br>Kparisero | 02 | 38 |
| 02-Savè | Kaboua | Kaboua, Okounfo, Alafia, Gogoro | 02 | 46 |
| 03- Kétou | Kétou center | Ketou center Odo -meta Idingni | 02 | 25 |
| 04-Agbangnizoun | Kinta | Kinta, Danhi, Ahissatogon | 02 | 36 |
| **Total** | **04 Boroughs** | **12 Villages** | **08 Interviews** | **145 people** |

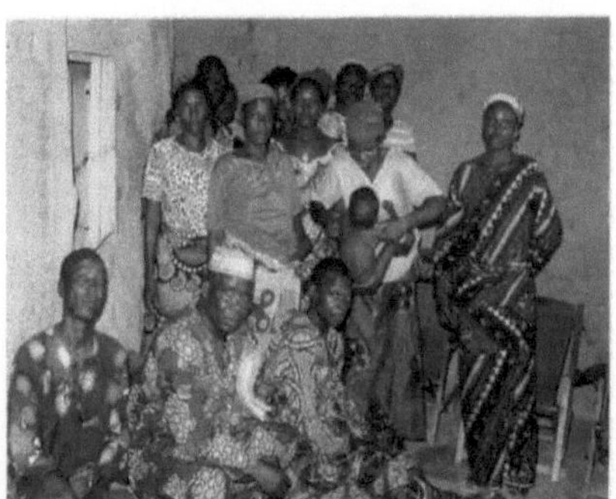

**Photo 9: A view taken at the end of an interview with patients and their carers at a traditional practitioner's in Kinta.**

(**Photo**: Claude MASSENON, March 2009).

Thus, at the end of the research, an interpretation framework was established, making it possible to structure the observations and testimonies gathered on the following essential aspects:

- the tradipratician's perception of the illness ;
- community beliefs ;
- examining the profile and socio-professional trajectory of grassroots communities;
- disease management by traditional healers ;
- the quality of traditional medicines ;
- building the capacity of traditional healers in the management of diseases ;
- information and communication on traditional medicine;
- traditional therapeutic methods ;
- the resources of traditional medicine ;
- collaboration between practitioners of both types of medicine;
- collaboration between traditional practitioners;
- the transmission of traditional therapeutic knowledge;
- protection of traditional therapeutic knowledge and know-how
- medicinal plants and flora of Benin ;
- the state of traditional medicines in Benin.

**3- Data processing and analysis**

Because of the dual nature of the data (qualitative and quantitative), the information was processed as follows:

**a) Manual processing of qualitative data**

The information transcribed on a notepad, the answers ticked off on the questionnaire and the results of the focus groups served as a basis for data analysis, using thematic grouping.

Data processing followed three stages: firstly, the constitution of thematic groups; secondly, the grouping of transcribed interviews by thematic group in the form of verbatims; and thirdly, the analysis and commentary of verbatims to serve as support for the writing of the thesis in the sense of the administration of evidence.

Thus, the following thematic groups from the interview and focus group transcripts were analyzed and commented on:

- Medicine's legal and institutional environment

  Traditional ;
- The foundations of the practice of traditional medicine ;
- Motives for using traditional medicine for health care needs ;
- Collaboration between traditional and modern medicine;

- Collaboration between traditional practitioners themselves;
- Traditional medicine and biodiversity ;
- Traditional medicine and source empowerment

  supply of plant materials ;
- Securing traditional healthcare services ;
- The qualification of traditional healers in the management of diseases ;
- Transmission of traditional therapeutic knowledge and skills;
- Protecting traditional knowledge ;
- Local traditional medicine industry.

**b) Computer processing of quantitative data**

A data entry mask was designed, and the data was entered and analyzed.

In addition, some cross-analyses were carried out to better appreciate the study variables within sub-groups and categories.

In the course of data collection, photography provided a significant data medium.

These data analysis and processing procedures generated indicators which also served as the basis for the results.

A number of difficulties arose during the course of the study.

**C- Difficulties encountered and approaches to solutions**

**1- Difficulties**

**a) Difficulties related to the scope of the study**

A study of traditional medicine is both a daring and delicate exercise, given the lack of an appropriate legislative and institutional framework for the practice of this medicine in Benin, and the individual and/or family nature of the transmission of endogenous knowledge and know-how.

**b) Difficulties in collecting data in the field**

The most apparent difficulties are linked to the scarcity of current documentation. Basic data are limited to an inventory of medicinal plants, and sometimes to the identification of their therapeutic virtues. Clinical and biological trials are not available, as they would be required to substantiate their scientific reliability.

Apart from these difficulties, there are others more specific to the sources of information, notably traditional practitioners and patients.

Indeed, in many cases, information is incomplete or deliberately truncated. The economy of truth is justified by the desire to protect traditional knowledge. It also reflects the ethnic and familial nature of endogenous traditional knowledge.

These are age-old practices linked to traditions, which in turn are linked to peoples. They are not always accessible to all but the initiated.

True traditional practitioners don't communicate very easily about their art.

Discretion is the order of the day in this field, which makes it difficult to gather data on traditional therapeutic methods.

Generally speaking, the period of memory required to obtain reliable information after illness is short-lived.

Moreover, in Traditional Medicine, the diagnosis of illness is not always precise. This is because the same individual interviewed may describe a variety of symptoms for one and the same disease, or different interpretations may be obtained from different people about a single condition.

Sometimes, people interpret different symptoms as illnesses.

As a result, in the case of death, for example, the cause is often not correctly established, and/or several causes may be associated in the traditional system.

**c) Difficulties linked to the lack of collaboration between practitioners of the two types of medicine**

The lack of formal collaboration between practitioners of traditional medicine and professionals of modern medicine poses the problem of materializing acts and facts such as, for example, the declaration of death following the failure of the tradipratician to treat an illness.

The lack of collaboration is a consequence of the lack of trust between the two types of healthcare actors, which justifies the lack of information on the evidence of progress made in the traditional medicine sub-sector.

**d) Difficulties in assessing the economic efficiency of traditional medicine.**

Analysis of the economic efficiency of traditional medicine is currently difficult in Africa in general, and in Benin in particular. The data often used is that of alternative or conventional medicine practiced in the West, or that of traditional medicine developed in Asia.

Practitioners of traditional African medicine in general, and of Beninese medicine in particular, have little or no education. Many have never attended school, which is why statistics are not kept.

In the absence of figures, it is virtually impossible to measure the contribution of this type of medicine to our countries' gross domestic product.

However, given that over 80% of the population use this treatment method for their healthcare needs, and that many of them recover their health, this contribution cannot be evaluated in monetary terms.

However, in terms of cost, treatment with traditional medicine is generally less expensive than the same treatment with conventional medicine.

Hence the economic efficiency of traditional medicine.

Certainly, economic efficiency is the dimension most often cited by practitioners and researchers alike to measure an organization's performance. Economic efficiency is expressed as the ratio between the quantity produced and the resources used to generate that production (Olivier de La Villarmois 2005).

In our countries, money matters are particularly sensitive. Questions about income and assets are distrusted. All those interviewed keep no accounts and make no tax declarations of their activities.

Traditional medicine is still practiced informally. This means that information on its economic efficiency is still unavailable.

### e) Institutional challenges

The institutional framework for the practice of traditional medicine in Benin is not conducive to the availability of the data needed for a better assessment of what has been achieved.

The national program for traditional pharmacopoeia and medicine, which acts as the institution responsible for translating the State's vision into policy, does not have enough skilled human resources to support it in drawing up action plans and strategic development plans.

No competent structure to respond to our concerns about the policy of integrating traditional medicine into the national health system; in particular with regard to :

- regulations ;
- research ;
- production of traditional medicines ;
- cooperation.

The coordinator, assisted by a single design manager (master's level), is responsible for the design, execution and supervision of more than ten thousand (10,000) tradipraticians.

### f) Difficulties in assessing the therapeutic efficacy of traditional remedies used by traditional practitioners

In the course of our fieldwork, we were unable to verify the clinical efficacy of traditional medicines offered by traditional practitioners in the treatment of the conditions listed in this study, due to a lack of documentation and, above all, the fact that this study is not oriented towards clinical trials.

Finally, the over-exploitation of flora in Benin, compounded by the perverse effects of illegal bushfires and climate change, has made it difficult to identify the medicinal plants cited for disease management in the various research zones.

In some cases, the tricks played by the various target populations have led to the dispersion of available resources and the ineffectiveness of our actions. For all these reasons, it is not easy to propose an exhaustive summary of our actions.

Notwithstanding all these difficulties, the research was carried out and the expected results were obtained, thanks to a number of circumstantial adjustments.

# PART TWO: RESULTS

## CHAPTER 3: REPERTOIRES OF COMMON ILLNESSES AND TRADITIONAL REMEDIES USED BY TRADITIONAL PRACTITIONERS TO TREAT THEM

### A- Common diseases in surveyed localities

#### 1- Statistical data on consultations in surveyed localities

a) In Kinta district (with a population of 6,000)

> **Kinta district monthly consultation statement for 2007.**

**Table 6:** Record of monthly consultations for 2007 at the Kinta district health center

| Pathologies Period | Palu | AD* - AD | Friends * | AGI* | STDS | Dia* | IRA* | LT* | LCA* | HTA* |
|---|---|---|---|---|---|---|---|---|---|---|
| January | 40 | 00 | 01 | 00 | 00 | 01 | 05 | 06 | 00 | 01 |
| February | 31 | 00 | 01 | 00 | 00 | 01 | 02 | 09 | 00 | 01 |
| March | 57 | 01 | 00 | 03 | 00 | 00 | 05 | 09 | 00 | 00 |
| April | 58 | 00 | 00 | 02 | 00 | 00 | 00 | 09 | 00 | 02 |
| May | 45 | 00 | 05 | 01 | 00 | 00 | 02 | 10 | 00 | 01 |
| June | 89 | 04 | 00 | 17 | 00 | 00 | 27 | 13 | 00 | 02 |
| July | 67 | 05 | 00 | 11 | 00 | 00 | 26 | 09 | 00 | 04 |
| August | 101 | 08 | 02 | 00 | 06 | 00 | 32 | 19 | 00 | 02 |
| September | 117 | 07 | 00 | 19 | 00 | 00 | 64 | 07 | 00 | 04 |
| October | 124 | 08 | 00 | 21 | 01 | 00 | 97 | 13 | 00 | 04 |
| November | 102 | 07 | 00 | 16 | 00 | 00 | 57 | 09 | 00 | 06 |
| December | 79 | 05 | 00 | 07 | 00 | 00 | 30 | 10 | 00 | 01 |
| **Total** | **910** | **45** | **09** | **97** | **07** | **02** | **347** | **123** | **00** | **28** |

**Table 7:** Presentation of the top five diseases most frequently observed at the Kinta district health center in 2007.

**NB:**

* *AD: Dermatological conditions*
* *Palu : Malaria*
* *AGI : Gastrointestinal disorders*
* *ARI : Acute respiratory infections*
* *LT : Trauma injuries*

**CVD : Cardiovascular disorders*
** HTA : Hypertension*
**ANEMIA: Anemia*
**DIA: Diarrhoea*

| Conditions | Number of consultations |
|---|---|
| 1 Malaria | 910 |
| 2 Acute respiratory infections | 347 |
| 3 Traumatic injuries | 123 |
| 4 Gastrointestinal disorders | 97 |
| 5 Dermatological conditions | 46 |
| **Total** | **1522** |

> **Monthly record of consultations at the Kinta district health center in 2008.**

**Table 8:** Record of monthly consultations for 2008 at the Kinta district health center.

| Pathologies Period | Malaria | AD | Friends | AGI | MST | Dia | IRA | LT | ACV | HTA |
|---|---|---|---|---|---|---|---|---|---|---|
| January | 70 | 02 | 00 | 17 | 00 | 00 | 52 | 05 | 04 | 00 |
| February | 81 | 01 | 10 | 32 | 02 | 00 | 39 | 08 | 00 | 01 |
| March | 65 | 10 | 04 | 16 | 01 | 00 | 23 | 00 | 00 | 14 |
| April | 93 | 03 | 14 | 16 | 00 | 00 | 25 | 11 | 00 | 04 |
| May | 105 | 10 | 21 | 32 | 00 | 00 | 51 | 13 | 00 | 03 |
| June | 146 | 07 | 26 | 32 | 00 | 00 | 49 | 02 | 00 | 00 |
| July | 85 | 05 | 14 | 27 | 01 | 01 | 34 | 04 | 01 | 02 |
| August | 70 | 01 | 10 | 12 | 00 | 00 | 32 | 10 | 00 | 00 |
| September | 69 | 02 | 13 | 08 | 01 | 00 | 29 | 10 | 00 | 01 |
| October | 85 | 07 | 04 | 14 | 00 | 02 | 33 | 07 | 00 | 01 |
| November | 98 | 11 | 12 | 23 | 00 | 12 | 50 | 07 | 00 | 03 |
| December | 52 | 09 | 03 | 19 | 04 | 00 | 30 | 06 | 00 | 02 |
| **Total** | **1019** | **68** | **131** | **248** | **09** | **15** | **447** | **83** | **05** | **31** |

**Table 9:** Presentation of the top five diseases most frequently observed at the Kinta district health center in 2008.

| Conditions | Number of consultations |
|---|---|
| 1 Malaria | 1019 |
| 2 Acute respiratory infections | 447 |
| 3 Gastrointestinal disorders | 248 |
| 4 Anemia | 131 |
| 5 Traumatic injuries | 83 |
| **Total** | **1888** |

a) In the arrondissement of Kétou-centre (with a population of 39,000)

> **2007 monthly consultation report from the Kétou commune health center.**

**Table 10**: Record of monthly consultations for 2007 at the Kétou health center

| Pathologies Period | Malaria | AD | Friends | AGI | MST | Dia | IRA | LT | ACV | HTA |
|---|---|---|---|---|---|---|---|---|---|---|
| January | 243 | 10 | 25 | 43 | 03 | 00 | 108 | 12 | 00 | 00 |
| February | 186 | 13 | 14 | 11 | 07 | 00 | 55 | 48 | 00 | 03 |
| March | 218 | 13 | 04 | 08 | 07 | 00 | 82 | 19 | 00 | 08 |
| April | 185 | 00 | 14 | 16 | 05 | 01 | 53 | 23 | 00 | 13 |
| May | 248 | 00 | 48 | 10 | 10 | 00 | 49 | 19 | 00 | 00 |
| June | 425 | 20 | 84 | 00 | 05 | 01 | 101 | 07 | 00 | 05 |
| July | 329 | 22 | 149 | 04 | 08 | 04 | 87 | 25 | 00 | 07 |
| August | 481 | 24 | 153 | 00 | 07 | 03 | 109 | 00 | 14 | 00 |
| September | 522 | 13 | 147 | 00 | 05 | 01 | 162 | 00 | 00 | 14 |
| October | 606 | 18 | 134 | 07 | 03 | 00 | 202 | 18 | 00 | 07 |
| November | - | - | - | - | - | - | - | - | - | - |
| December | - | - | - | - | - | - | - | - | - | - |
| **Total** | **3443** | **143** | **772** | **99** | **60** | **10** | **1008** | **171** | **00** | **71** |

**Table 11:** Presentation of the top five most frequently reported diseases at the Kétou commune health center in 2007.

| Conditions | Number of consultations |
|---|---|
| 1 Malaria | 3643 |
| 2 Acute respiratory infections | 1008 |
| 3 Traumatic injuries | 772 |
| 4 Gastrointestinal disorders | 171 |
| 5 Dermatological conditions | 143 |
| **Total** | **5565** |

> **2008 monthly consultation report from the Kétou commune health center.**

**Table 12**: Record of monthly consultations for 2008 at the Kétou health center

| Pathologies Period | Malaria | AD | Friends | AGI | MST | Dia | IRA | LT | ACV | HTA |
|---|---|---|---|---|---|---|---|---|---|---|
| January | 290 | 00 | 26 | 00 | 15 | 12 | 105 | 31 | 00 | 09 |
| February | 214 | 00 | 17 | 00 | 07 | 06 | 54 | 41 | 00 | 07 |
| March | 182 | 13 | 14 | 00 | 00 | 07 | 39 | 68 | 00 | 08 |
| April | 265 | 00 | 17 | 00 | 00 | 07 | 80 | 45 | 00 | 14 |
| May | 285 | 00 | 36 | 00 | 04 | 08 | 56 | 49 | 00 | 08 |
| June | 395 | 00 | 56 | 00 | 05 | 09 | 84 | 62 | 00 | 09 |
| July | 606 | 48 | 120 | 47 | 00 | 00 | 101 | 95 | 00 | 11 |
| August | 451 | 25 | 65 | 49 | 05 | 14 | 75 | 25 | 00 | 03 |
| September | 602 | 22 | 120 | 48 | 00 | 08 | 88 | 47 | 00 | 04 |
| October | 689 | 26 | 66 | 56 | 09 | 17 | 212 | 47 | 01 | 07 |
| November | 997 | 18 | 76 | 63 | 12 | 00 | 176 | 39 | 00 | 14 |
| December | 335 | 24 | 49 | 92 | 21 | 00 | 62 | 37 | 01 | 06 |
| **Total** | **4912** | **166** | **661** | **395** | **76** | **88** | **1113** | **586** | **02** | **100** |

**Table 14:** Presentation of the top five most-reported diseases at the Kétou health center in 2008.

| Conditions | Number of consultations |
|---|---|
| 1 Malaria | 4912 |
| 2 Acute respiratory infections | 1113 |
| 3 Anemia | 661 |
| 4 Traumatic injuries | 586 |
| 5 Gastrointestinal disorders | 395 |
| **Total** | **7667** |

b) In the Kaboua district (with a population of 7,000)

> **Record of monthly consultations for 2007 at the Kaboua district health center.**

**Table 15**: Record of monthly consultations for 2007 at the Kaboua district health center

| Pathologies Period | Malaria | AD | Friends | AGI | MST | Dia | IRA | LT | ACV | HTA |
|---|---|---|---|---|---|---|---|---|---|---|
| January | 18 | 00 | 00 | 02 | 00 | 02 | 12 | 01 | 00 | 00 |
| February | 10 | 01 | 00 | 00 | 00 | 08 | 01 | 02 | 00 | 01 |
| March | 33 | 04 | 01 | 04 | 00 | 02 | 04 | 03 | 00 | 00 |
| April | 09 | 00 | 00 | 00 | 00 | 01 | 01 | 02 | 00 | 00 |
| May | 27 | 03 | 00 | 03 | 00 | 05 | 05 | 08 | 00 | 00 |
| June | ND | ND | ND | ND | ND | ND | ND | ND | ND | ND |
| July | 46 | 02 | 02 | 00 | 00 | 13 | 13 | 03 | 00 | 01 |
| August | 68 | 00 | 00 | 04 | 00 | 19 | 19 | 07 | 00 | 00 |
| September | 71 | 01 | 00 | 00 | 00 | 29 | 29 | 01 | 00 | 00 |
| October | 66 | 00 | 00 | 00 | 00 | 29 | 29 | 02 | 00 | 00 |
| November | 57 | 01 | 00 | 05 | 00 | 19 | 19 | 06 | 00 | 03 |

| December | 27 | 02 | 00 | 02 | 00 | 13 | 13 | 02 | 00 | 01 |
|---|---|---|---|---|---|---|---|---|---|---|
| **Total** | **432** | **14** | **03** | **20** | **00** | **140** | **145** | **37** | **00** | **06** |

ND : Not available

**Table 16**: Presentation of the top five diseases most frequently reported in consultations at the Kaboua district health center in 2007.

| Conditions | Number of consultations |
|---|---|
| 1 Malaria | 432 |
| 2 Acute respiratory infections | 145 |
| 3 Traumatic injuries | 140 |
| 4 Gastrointestinal disorders | 37 |
| 5 Dermatological conditions | 20 |
| **Total** | **774** |

**Table 17**: Record of monthly consultations for 2008 at the Kaboua district health center

| Pathologies Period | Malaria | AD | Friends | AGI | MST | Dia | IRA | LT | ACV | HTA |
|---|---|---|---|---|---|---|---|---|---|---|
| January | 32 | 00 | 00 | 08 | 00 | 10 | 26 | 00 | 00 | 00 |
| February | 32 | 01 | 00 | 02 | 00 | 08 | 10 | 03 | 00 | 00 |
| March | 20 | 01 | 00 | 04 | 00 | 04 | 08 | 05 | 01 | 00 |
| April | 21 | 00 | 00 | 04 | 00 | 03 | 04 | 00 | 00 | 02 |
| May | 39 | 00 | 00 | 07 | 00 | 04 | 08 | 05 | 00 | 01 |
| June | 37 | 04 | 00 | 07 | 00 | 04 | 03 | 03 | 00 | 01 |
| July | ND | ND | ND | ND | ND | ND | ND | ND | ND | ND |
| August | 28 | 00 | 00 | 02 | 00 | 01 | 05 | 03 | 00 | 00 |
| September | 44 | 00 | 00 | 00 | 00 | 03 | 24 | 02 | 00 | 01 |
| October | 39 | 00 | 00 | 00 | 00 | 05 | 21 | 05 | 00 | 04 |
| November | 39 | 00 | 00 | 01 | 00 | 06 | 07 | 02 | 00 | 00 |
| December | 34 | 00 | 00 | 00 | 00 | 09 | 06 | 03 | 00 | 03 |
| **Total** | **365** | **06** | **00** | **35** | **00** | **24** | **122** | **31** | **01** | **13** |

**Table 18**: Presentation of the top five diseases most frequently reported in consultations at the Kaboua district health center in 2008.

| Conditions | Number of consultations |
|---|---|
| 1 Malaria | 365 |
| 2 Acute respiratory infections | 122 |
| 3 Gastrointestinal disorders | 35 |
| 4 Traumatic injuries | 31 |
| | 24 |
| 5 Diarrhea | |
| **Total** | **577** |

c) In the Nikki - Centre district (with a population of 99,000)

> **Record of monthly consultations for 2007 at the Nikki commune health center.**

**Table 19**: Record of monthly consultations for 2007 at the Nikki- Centre district health center

| Pathologies Period | Malaria | AD | Friends | AGI | MST | Dia | IRA | LT | ACV | HTA |
|---|---|---|---|---|---|---|---|---|---|---|
| January | 719 | 12 | 90 | 184 | 12 | 114 | - | - | 04 | 01 |
| February | 708 | 32 | 63 | 146 | 20 | 95 | - | 01 | 04 | - |
| March | 818 | 41 | 60 | 219 | 24 | 108 | 07 | 07 | 03 | - |
| April | 734 | 44 | 50 | 220 | 21 | 110 | 07 | 08 | 05 | 03 |
| May | 1188 | 63 | 88 | 224 | 11 | 230 | 05 | 08 | 05 | 03 |
| June | 1786 | 39 | 82 | 304 | 15 | 131 | 13 | 06 | 05 | - |
| July | 1518 | 45 | 132 | 189 | 10 | 140 | 04 | 07 | 06 | - |
| August | 1312 | 31 | 82 | 188 | 14 | 107 | 03 | 03 | 04 | - |
| September | 1899 | 38 | 180 | 293 | 23 | 166 | 08 | 08 | 02 | - |
| October | 2597 | 44 | 175 | 411 | 18 | 276 | 06 | 08 | 04 | 05 |
| November | 2321 | 32 | 208 | 301 | 26 | 299 | 10 | 13 | 02 | 01 |
| December | 1324 | 21 | 235 | 342 | 19 | 239 | 04 | 16 | 02 | 01 |
| **Total** | **16836** | **442** | **1440** | **2514** | **213** | **2003** | **54** | **65** | **41** | **14** |

**Table 20:** Presentation of the top five most frequently notified diseases at the Nikki - center district health center in 2007.

| Conditions | Number of cases |
|---|---|
| 1 Malaria | 16 836 |
| 2 Acute respiratory infections | 2512 |
| 3 Diarrhea | 2003 |
| 4 Anemia | 1440 |
| 5 Dermatological conditions | 442 |
| **Total** | **23235** |

**Table 21**: Record of monthly consultations for 2008 at the Nikki -centre district health center

| Pathologies Period | Malaria | AD | Friends | AGI | MST | Dia | IRA | LT | ACV | HTA |
|---|---|---|---|---|---|---|---|---|---|---|
| January | 1095 | 48 | 38 | 187 | 11 | 106 | 445 | 202 | 02 | 09 |
| February | 1129 | 39 | 55 | 234 | 06 | 31 | 443 | 179 | 01 | 09 |
| March | 1356 | 44 | 44 | 322 | 10 | 202 | 490 | 201 | 01 | 05 |
| April | 1192 | 61 | 49 | 261 | 14 | 157 | 100 | 207 | 03 | 06 |
| May | 1310 | 63 | 101 | 195 | 11 | 143 | 230 | 205 | - | 10 |
| June | 2613 | 68 | 282 | 337 | 04 | 223 | 225 | 202 | - | 12 |
| July | 2349 | 57 | 282 | 251 | 12 | 152 | 218 | 169 | 01 | 08 |
| August | 2313 | 30 | 196 | 185 | 04 | 117 | 194 | 139 | - | 03 |
| September | 2173 | 53 | 186 | 306 | 04 | 235 | 166 | 136 | - | 09 |
| October | 2228 | 52 | 168 | 357 | 27 | 110 | 337 | 157 | - | 08 |
| November | 2361 | 49 | 129 | 408 | 16 | 187 | 292 | 97 | - | 16 |
| December | 1607 | 35 | 91 | 767 | 21 | 604 | 353 | 257 | - | 16 |
| **Total** | **19576** | **599** | **1348** | **3695** | **124** | **2345** | **3503** | **1886** | **08** | **144** |

**Table 22**: Presentation of the top five most frequently reported illnesses at the Nikki-

Centre health center in 2008.

| Conditions | Number of consultations |
|---|---|
| 1 Malaria | 18576 |
| 2 AGI | 3695 |
| 3 IRA | 3503 |
| 4 Diarrhea | 2345 |
| 5 Trauma lesions | 1886 |
| **Total** | **31005** |

To enable us to monitor trends in the various diseases over the two years, we present in a single table the annual records of the consultations most frequently encountered in the health facilities of the four study zones.

## 2- General epidemiological situation in the four areas surveyed

**Table 23**: Annual survey of consultations in the four survey areas

| Periods | Pathology<br>Locations | Palu | AD | Anemia | AGI | MST | DIA | IRA | Trauma | RVC | HTA |
|---|---|---|---|---|---|---|---|---|---|---|---|
| 2007 | Kinta | 910 | 45 | 09 | 97 | 07 | 02 | 347 | 123 | 00 | 28 |
| | Kétou | 3443 | 143 | 772 | 99 | 60 | 10 | 1.008 | 171 | 00 | 71 |
| | Kaboua | 432 | 14 | 03 | 20 | 00 | 140 | 145 | 37 | 00 | 06 |
| | Nikki | 16.836 | 442 | 1.440 | 2.514 | 213 | 2.003 | 54 | 65 | 41 | 14 |
| | **TOTAL I** | **21.621** | **644** | **2.224** | **2.730** | **280** | **2.155** | **1.554** | **396** | **41** | **119** |
| 2008 | Kinta | 1.019 | 67 | 131 | 248 | 09 | 15 | 407 | 83 | 05 | 31 |
| | Kétou | 4.019 | 166 | 661 | 355 | 76 | 88 | 1.113 | 586 | 02 | 100 |
| | Kaboua | 345 | 06 | 00 | 35 | 00 | 24 | 31 | 122 | 31 | 13 |
| | Nikki | 19.576 | 599 | 1.348 | 3.645 | 124 | 2.345 | 3.503 | 1.886 | 08 | 144 |
| | **TOTAL II** | **24.959** | **838** | **2.140** | **4.283** | **209** | **2.472** | **5.054** | **2.677** | **46** | **288** |

A number of observations can be made about the epidemiological situation in the four research sectors over the two reference years (2007 and 2008):

- malaria is numerically the leading cause of consultation in all four health centers surveyed
- The other four diseases are, in order:
  - gastrointestinal disorders(AGI);
  - acute respiratory infections (ARI);
  - diarrhea (DIA);
  - anemia (AMIES).

Over the two years, the Nikki- Centre arrondissement had the highest malaria prevalence rate (78.17%), making it a high malaria-propagation zone in Benin.

**B- Traditional remedies used by traditional practitioners to treat common illnesses**

**1- Malaria**

This study appears important in that it could serve as a benchmark in the choice of research programs on traditional remedies to improve the contribution of traditional medicine to improving access to healthcare in Benin.

In the present study, a repertory of remedies used in the management of diseases has been compiled, while the identification of medicinal plants used in the preparation of these remedies has been made possible.

***a) At the Kinta fon***

Plant used :
Scientific name: **SPONDIAS mombin Linn. (Anacardiaceae)**
French name: Mombin ou prune icaque
Directions for use : Drink a decoction of the plant's fresh leaves three times a day in a full beer glass.

***b) Among the Nago of Kétou***

Scientific name: **FAGARA xalanthoxyloïdes and HYMENOCARDIA acida Tull (Euphorbiaceae).**

French name caïlcédrat (fagara) and hymenocardia acida tull

Name in local language (Yoruba): Igui ata and igui orukpa.

Preparation: Dry the bark of the two plants and grind to a powder.

Directions for use : Drink one teaspoonful with warm porridge in a coffee cup.

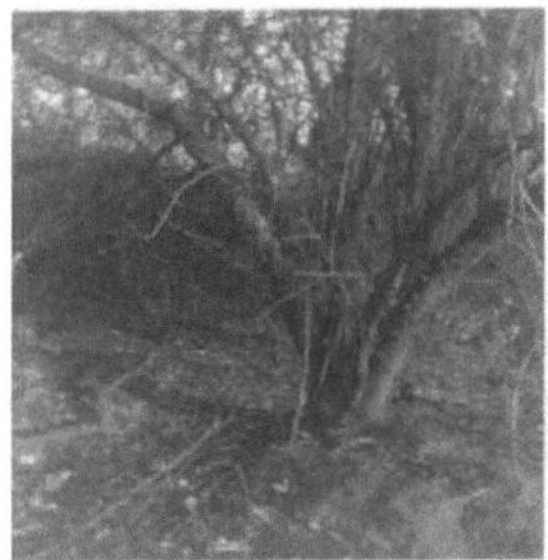

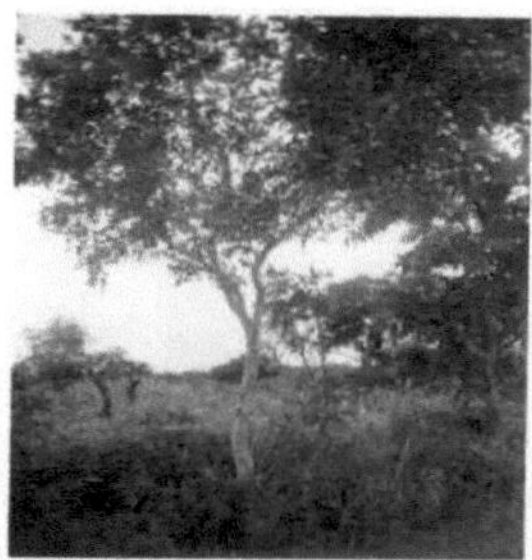

**Photo 10: FAGARA xalanthoxyloides and HYMENOCARDIA acida Tull (Photo Tiamiou AKPONNE, April 2009)**

Both plants are used in combination to treat malaria in the Nago environment of Kétou.

***c) Among the Nago of Savè***

Plant used
Scientific name: **CASSIA alata Linn**. (Cesalpiniaceae)
French appellation : Dartrier
Local language: asson
Preparation: Harvest the yellow flowers, dry them and grind them into powder. Use: Drink a teaspoonful of powder in a cup of lukewarm porridge, morning and evening, for a week.

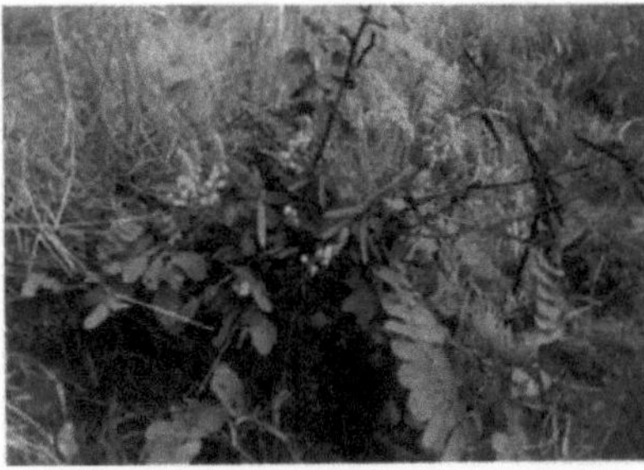

**Photo 11**: **CASSIA alata Linseed (Cesalpiniaceae).** Used to treat malaria in the Nago area of Savè **(Photo: Tiamiou AKPONNE, December 2009).**

### *d) The Nikki Bariba*

Plant used :
Scientific name: PTEROCARPUS **erinaceus Poir**
French appellation **:** Palisandre de Sénégal
In the local Bariba language: Tona or boutombou
En fon : Kosso
In Nago from Savè: Aïkpé
Directions for use : The decoction of leaves taken as inhalations, baths and drinks two or three times a day is a remedy against malaria.
The Nikki Bariba also use other plants in their drinks:

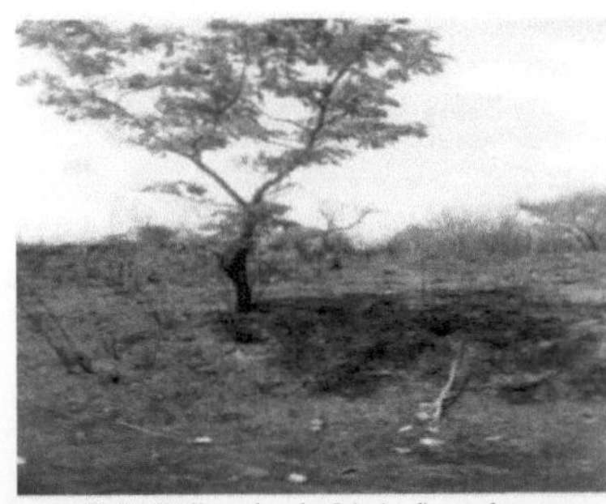

**Photo 12**: **PTEROCARPUS erinaceus Poir** (Palisandre du Sénégal) used to treat malaria in Nikki **(Photo Tiamiou AKPONNE, February 2010).**

Among the Bariba, Nago (Savè and Kétou), the dried leaves and bark of the mango tree are used as a decoction to treat malaria.
Plant used :
Zoological Name: **MANGNIFERA indica Linn**
French designation: Manguier
Name in local Bariba language: Mangodanrou
Properties and uses :

One glass of bamboo bark decoction taken three times a day is used to treat malaria.

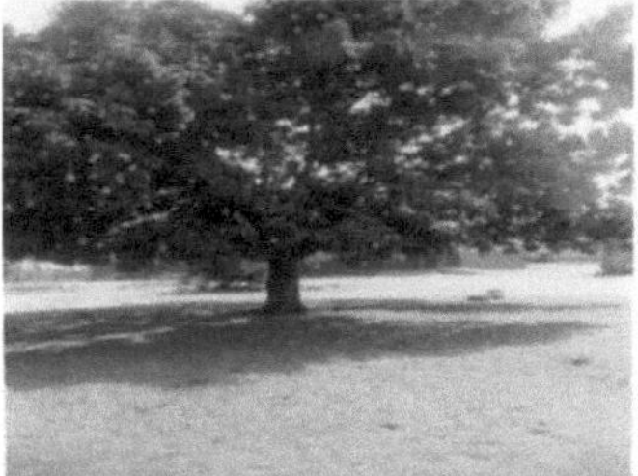

**Photo 13: MANGNIFERA indica** (mango tree. Used in Bariba environments to treat malaria. (**Photo Tiamiou AKPONNE, February 2010)**

## 2- Gastrointestinal disorders

### *a) At the Kinta fon*

Plant used :
Zoological Name: **OCINUM gratissimum Linn (Lamiaceae)**
French name: Plante moustique ou buisson thé ou feuille fièvre
Local Fon name: Tchayo
Preparation and directions for use: Triturate a handful of leaves in a liter of drinking water to collect the filtrate.

In the same treatment, the sauce or vegetable leaves of the plant are recommended in place of the filtra.

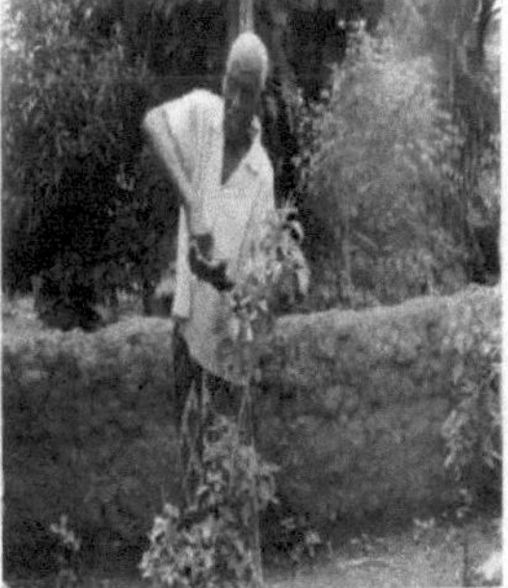

**Photo 14**: A traditional practitioner from Wèdjè (Kinta) passes on his therapeutic knowledge of the **OCINUM gratissimum Linn** plant (mosquito plant), used to treat gastrointestinal ailments.

**(Photo Claude MASSENON, March 2009**).

### *b) Among the Nago of Kétou*

Plant used :
Scientific name: **PSIDIUM guajava Linn. (Myrtaceae)**
Appellation Française : Guava tree
Name in local Nago language: Igui Chinkoun
Preparation: a decoction of the leaves of this plant and a piece of Kaolin. Directions for use : take three (03) times a day, morning, noon and evening, in a full beer glass.

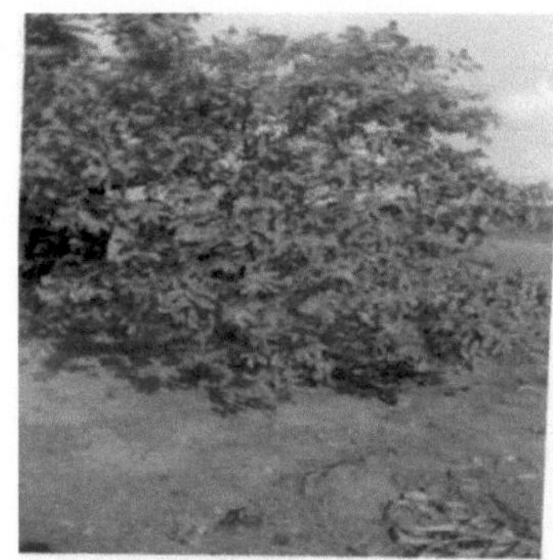

**Photo 15**: **PSIDIUM guajava Linn** (Guava tree) used in the Nago environment of Kétou to treat dysentery **(Photo: Tiamiou AKPONNE, April 2009).**

### *c) Among the Nago of Savè*

Plant used :
Zoological Name: **ANNONA senegalensis Pers (Annonaceae)**
Appellation Française : Pomme Cannelle du Sénégal, annone
Nago local language name: Ambo.
Preparation: Aqueous macerate of stem bark or leafy twigs is anti-diarrheal and anti-dysenteric.
Uses : Drink a glass of beer 3 times a day (morning, noon and evening) until cured.

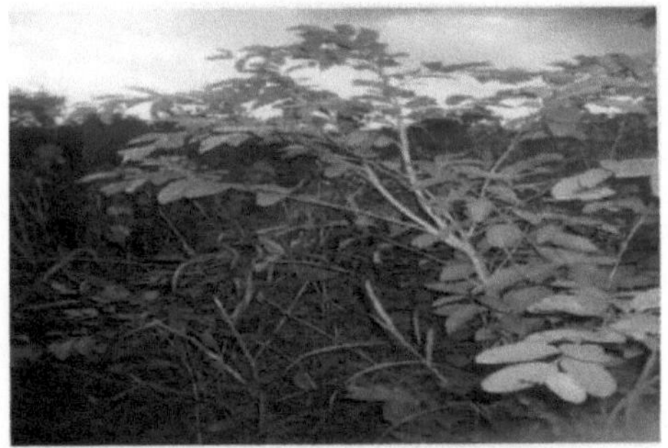

**Photo 16**: **ANNONA senegalensis Pers(Annonaceae)**, also known as annone. Used in the Nago environment of Savè to treat dysentery.

**(Photo Tiamiou AKPONNE, December 2009)**

### *d) Among the Bariba of Nikki*

Plant :
Zoological Name: **MUSA paradisiaca Linn (Musaceae)**
French name: Bananier
Name in local Bariba language: Aguèdèkorou
Directions for use: Banana pulp decoction is used to treat severe childhood diarrhoea; one tablespoonful twice a day (morning and evening).

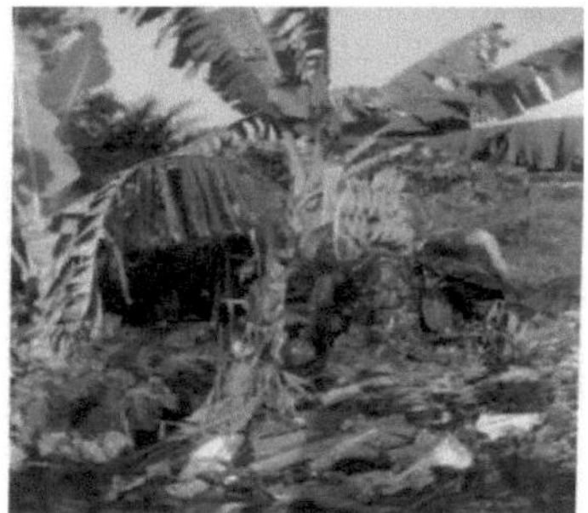

Photo 17: **MUSA paradisiaca Linn** (banana tree) used to treat infantile diarrhoea
**(Photo: Tiamiou AKPONNE, February 2010)**

Plant used:
Zoological Name: **SWIETENIA senegalensis A.Juas (Meliaceae)**
French designation: Acajou du Sénégal or Caïlcédrat or Quinquina du Sénégal
Local Bariba name: Biribou or bilibou
Preparation and directions for use

The decoction of the bark is used as a drink at a rate of half a beer glass three (03) times a day (morning, noon and evening).

One teaspoonful of dried trunk bark powder is diluted in a teacup of lukewarm water and drunk as coffee twice a day (morning and evening). It has multiple therapeutic functions.

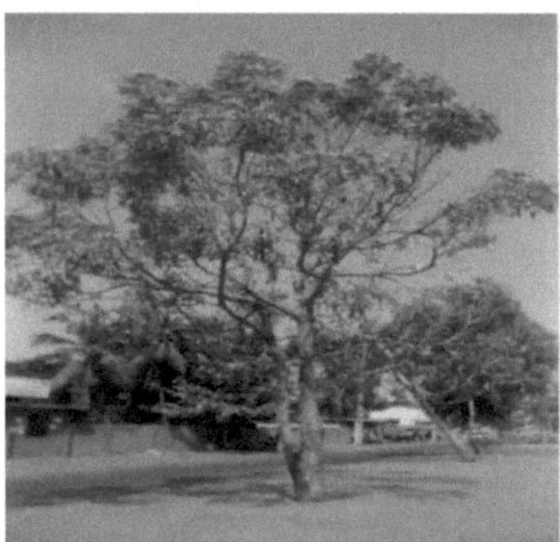

**Photo 18**: **SWIETENIA senegalensis A. Juas** (Senegalese Quinquina plant or Senegalese Mahogany) used to treat gastrointestinal ailments in Bariba environments **(Photo: Tiamiou AKPONNE, February 2010).**

### 3- Acute respiratory infections: bronchitis

### *a) The Fon of Kinta*

Plant used :
Zoological Name: **CALOTROPIS procera Ait. (Asclepiadaceae)**
French name: Arbre à soie du Sénégal or pomme de Sodome or herbe hirondelle
Name in the local Fongbé language: Kpinto or Wagachiman Preparation: Decoction of five (05) to six (06) leaves of the plant. A small piece of shea butter is added to the decoction.

Directions for use : One tablespoon for children and one liqueur glass for adults three (03) times a day (morning, noon and evening).

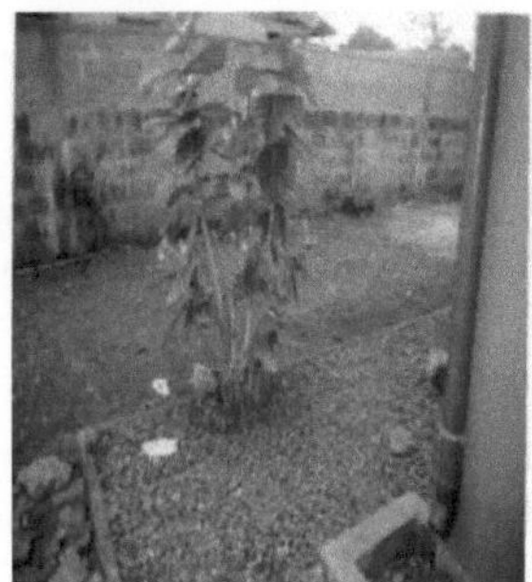

**Photo 19: CALOTROPIS procera Ait** (Senegalese silk tree or Sodom apple or swallow grass). Used to treat bronchitis in Fon

**(Photo: Tiamiou AKPONNE, March 2009).**

### *b) Among the Nago of Kétou*

Plant used:

Zoological Name: **DANIELLA thurifera**

French name: Térébenthe ou copalier africain de Balsam

Synonym: B. micrantha

In the local Nago language: Ira or Ouya

Preparation and directions for use: Leaf decoction is a cough sedative for children. Drink one tablespoonful 3 times a day (morning, noon and evening) until cured.

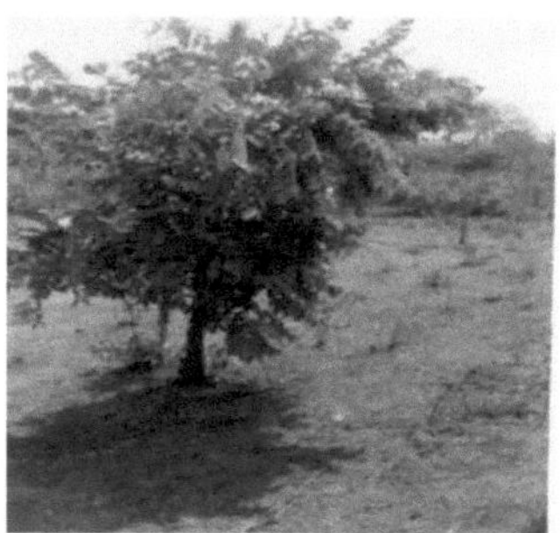

**Photo 20**: **DANIELLA thurifera** (Terebenthe or African Balsam copal) used to treat acute respiratory infections.

**(Photo: Tiamiou AKPONNE, February 2010)**

### *c) Among the Nago of Savè*

Plant used :

Zoological Name: **BORASSUS aethiopum Mart (Arecaceae)**

French appellation : Rônier

Name in local language: Agbon gbodjoï

Preparation and directions for use : A decoction of the roots of young shoots is used to treat sore throats, bronchitis and hoarseness. Drink a glass of Bamboo twice (02) a day (morning and evening).

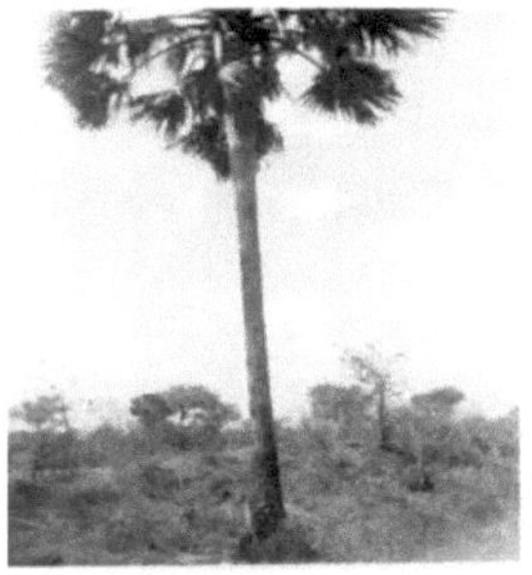

**Photo 21**: **BORASSUS aethiopum Mart** (Rônier) used to treat bronchitis in the Nago area of Savè.

**(Photo Tiamiou AKPONNE, December 2009)**

### *d) Among the Bariba of Nikki*

The **SWIETENIA senegalensis** plant, whose bark is used to treat gastrointestinal infections, is also used to treat acute respiratory infections (bronchitis).

Plant used:

Zoological Name: **SWIETENIA senegalensis A. Juas**

French appellation: Acajou du Sénégal or Caïlcédrat or Quinquina du Sénégal.

Local Bariba name: Bilibou or bilibou

Preparation Directions for use: The powder from the dried bark of the trunk is diluted at a rate of one teaspoonful in a teacup of lukewarm water and drunk as coffee twice a day (morning and evening). The same powder can be diluted in an alcoholic beverage. Drink half a glass of liqueur once a day for at least 7 days.

**4- Anemia**

***a) The Fon of Kinta***

Plant used:

Zoological Name: **BASELLA rubra**

Appellation Française: Baselle blanche

Name in local Fon language: Djomakou

Preparation: A decoction of the plant is indicated as a tonic for anemia.

Directions for use : One bamboo glass of the solution morning, noon and night for the duration of the treatment.

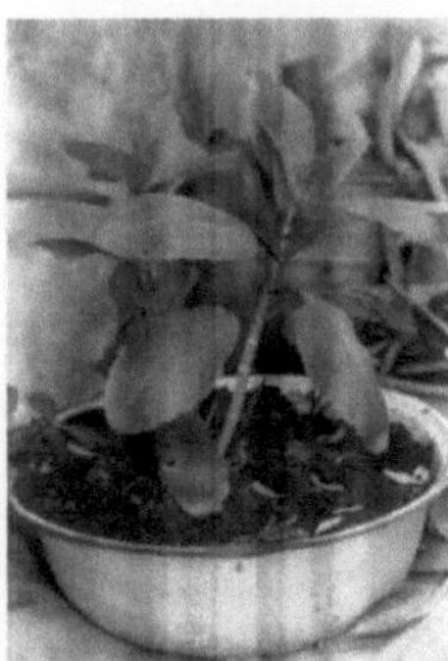

**Photo 22: BASELLA**
Kinta in treatment

**Tiamiou AKPONNE, March**

**rubra** used in anemia therapy as a restorative.

**(Photo,2009)**

### *b) Among the Nago of Kétou*

Plant used:

Zoological Name: CODATUM sorghum coloran

French appellation :

Nago local language name: Ipo- onin

Preparation: Herb decoction

Directions for use : Drink one 250ml bamboo glass 3 times a day (morning, noon, evening) for three to five days.

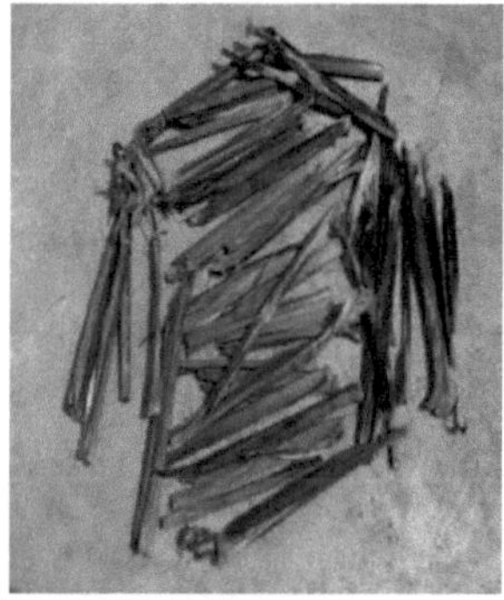

**Photo 23**: CODATUM sorghum coloran herb used to treat anemia in the Nago environment of Kétou **(Photo: Bolivar -Photo, April 2009)**

### *c) Among the Nago of Savè*

Plant used:

Zoological Name: **JATROPHA gossypiifolia red medicinal plant**

Appellation Française : Poughère (red)

Name in local Nago language: Opopo -hu pupa

Preparation: Decoction of a small quantity of plant leaves.

Directions for use : One bamboo glass three (03) times a day (morning, noon and evening) for one week.

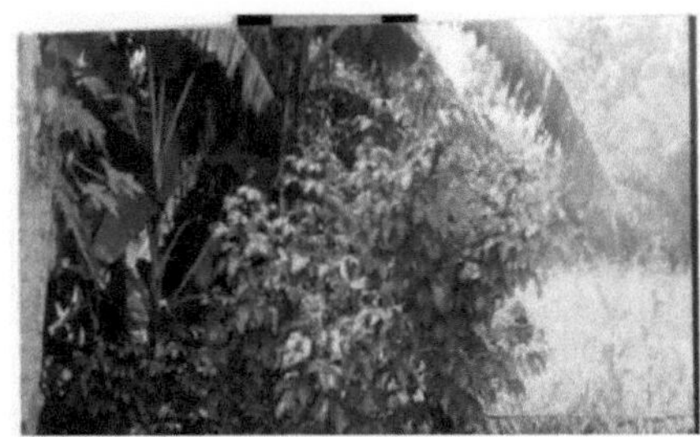

Photo 24: **JATROPHA gossypiifolia, a red medicinal plant** used to treat anemia in the Nago area of Savè.

**(Photo: Tiamiou AKPONNE, December 2009)**

### *d) Among the Bariba of Nikki*

Among other remedies, the Bariba use the following traditional plant-based medicine to treat anemia:

Plant used:

Zoological Name: **PARKIA biglobosa Benth (Mimosaceae)**

French name: Mimosa pourpre or arbre à fauve.

In Benin, it is commonly known as néré or nété.

Local name: in Bariba, it is called donm

Directions for use : Decocted leaf juice is used as a drink, at the rate of one beer glass 3 times a day (morning, noon and evening).

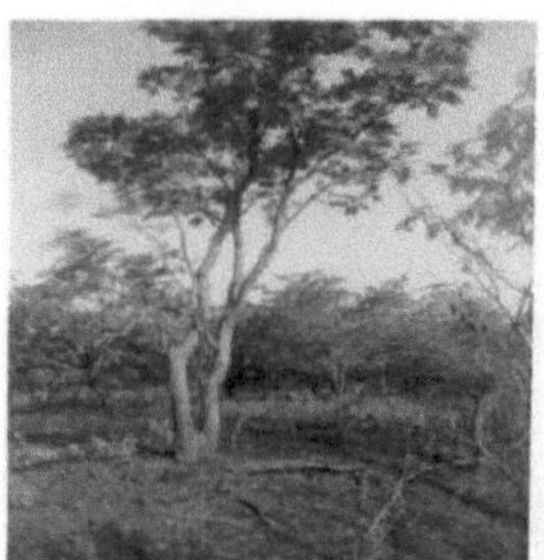

Photo 25: **PARKIA biglobosa Benth** (already identified) in French néré or nété. Used in Bariba environments to treat anemia, the trunk bark and roots in decoction treat sterility and venereal diseases.

**(Photo: Tiamiou AKPONNE, February 2010)**

## 5- Traumatic injuries

### *a) The Fon of Kinta*

Plant used :

Zoological Name: FAGARA Xanthoxyloides

French name : **Caïlcédrat**

Name in local language: Hètin

Properties and uses: Root powder is used as a toothpaste in the treatment of toothache. The roots are also used as toothpicks in the treatment of dental caries.

### *b) Among the Nago of Kétou*

Plant used :

Scientific name: **HYMENOCARDI acida tull (Euphorbiaceae).**

Name in local language: Igui Okpa or igui ossoun

Properties and directions for use : Take one glass of bamboo root decoction three times a day (morning, noon and evening) to treat traumatic gastric ulcer lesions.

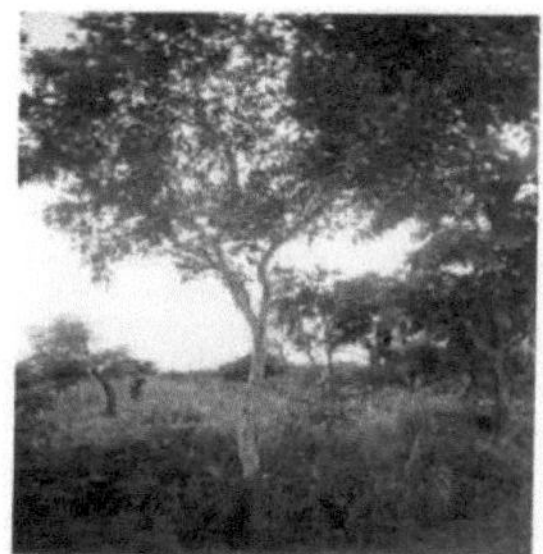

Plant already identified: **HYMENOCARDI acida tull** (Euphorbiaceae) indicated for the treatment of traumatic lesions in the Nago environment of Kétou.
**(Photo: Tiamiou AKPONNE, April 2009)**

### *c) Among the Nago of Savè*

Plant used

Zoological Name: Butyrospermes paradoxum

French name: Karité

Local name: Egui èmin

Properties and instructions for use :

- The decoction from the bark of the trunk is used as a drink in three bamboo glasses three times a day (morning, noon and evening) to treat internal trauma.
- The fatty substance from the seeds, called shea butter, is used for sprains, cosmetics and dermatosis.

### *d) Among the Bariba of Nikki*

Plant used:
Zoological Name: Swietenia Senegalensis
French appellation: Acajou du Sénégal or Caïlcédrat or Quinquina du Sénégal.

Local Bariba name: Bilibou or bilibou

Preparation and directions for use: Dried trunk bark powder is diluted to a teaspoonful in a teacup of lukewarm water and drunk as coffee twice a day (morning and evening). The same powder can be diluted in an alcoholic beverage. Drink half a glass of liqueur once a day for at least 7 days.

**Table 24:** Overview of traditional remedies proposed for the treatment of the five diseases in the various localities

| Locations / Diseases''''^ | Kinta | **Kétou** | **Kaboua** | **Nikki** | **Comments** |
|---|---|---|---|---|---|
| **Malaria** | Decocted leaves of: Spondias mombin Linn (Mombin or icaque plum) taken as a drink at the rate of one glass three times a day treats malaria. | Drink one teaspoonful of the powdered dried bark of fagara Xanthoxyloid plants and hymenocardia acida tull in a small coffee cup with lukewarm porridge. | Drink a teaspoonful, half-full, of the powdered dried flowers of the cassia alata linseed plant (Dartier) in lukewarm porridge. | Use the decoction of Pterocarpus erinaceus Poir leaves in inhalations, baths and drinks two to three times a day for at least one week. | **No agreement (treatments differ from one locality to another)** |
| **Gastrointestinal disorders** | Powder of the dried bark of the fagara plants Xanthoxyloïdes and hymenocardia acida tull taken at a rate of one teaspoonful in water or in any other solution treats malaria. | Gardenia erubescens bark decoction or macerate, taken as a drink at the rate of one glass three times a day, treats gastrointestinal disorders. | Daniella thurifera leaf decoction, taken at a rate of one tablespoon three times a day until cured, is a cough sedative for children. | The dried bark powder of K haya Senegalensis (Senegalese mahogany, or caïlcédrat), known in the local language as Nago aganho, in Fon as Zounza and in Bariba as biribou, taken as a drink at the rate of one cup every morning, treats trauma. | No agreement |
| **Gastrointestinal disorders** | Drink in a beer glass the filtrate of five to six Ocinum gratissimum Linn leaves crushed in a liter of drinking water three times a day for two days. | Drink the decoction of Psidium quajava Linn leaves prepared with a piece of kaolin three times a day morning, noon and night in a full beer glass. | Aqueous macerate of annona senegalensis Pero stem bark or leafy twigs, drunk in a beer glass three (03) times a day until cured, is a remedy for gastrointestinal ailments. | Banana pulp decoctate is used to treat severe infantile diarrhea; one tablespoonful twice a day for a week. | No agreement |
| **Acute respiratory infections: bronchitis** | Decoction of five (05) to six (06) leaves of the Calotropies procera Ait plant plus a small piece of shea butter taken as a drink at a rate of one tablespoon for children and one small liqueur glass for adults three times a day (morning, noon and evening). | Daniella thurifera leaf decoction is a cough sedative for children, taken in one tablespoon three times a day (morning, noon and evening) until cured. | Borassus aethiopum Mart root decoction taken as a drink in a bamboo glass twice (02) a day treats hoarseness of the voice. | Powdered dried bark from the trunk of the Swietenia plant. senegalensis diluted in a teaspoonful of lukewarm water taken twice (02) a day (morning and evening) treats bronchitis. The same amount of powder diluted in an alcoholic beverage at | No agreement |

| | and evening) treat bronchitis | | | Half a glass of liqueur taken once a day for at least seven (07) days also treats bronchitis in adults. | |
|---|---|---|---|---|---|
| **Anemia** | A decoction of six (06) to eight (08) Basella rubra leaves taken as a drink in a bamboo glass three (03) times a day treats anemia. | The decoction of a tuft of Codatum sorghum coloran, known in the local language as Nago de Kétou Ipo-onin, taken as a drink at the rate of one beer glass three times a day for three days, treats anemia. | The decoction or macerated leaf of red medicinal Jatropha Gossypiifolia taken as a drink in a bamboo glass three (03) times a day for a week is restorative for anemia. | In Bariba country, the decoction of the leaves of the Parkia biglobosa Benth plant, known in the local language as donm, is used to treat anemia, taken as a drink of one beer glass three times a day for at least a week. | No agreement |
| **Traumatic injuries** | Fagara Xanthoxyloid root powder is used in the treatment of toothache as a toothpaste. The roots are also used as toothpicks in the treatment of dental caries. | The decoction of hymenocardia acida tull roots taken as a drink in a bamboo glass three times a day (morning, noon and evening) treats traumatic gastric ulcer lesions. | The decoction of Butyrospermes paradoxum trunk bark is used as a drink in three bamboo glasses three times a day (morning, noon and evening) to treat internal trauma. The fatty substance in the seeds, known as shea butter, is used for sprains, cosmetics and dermatosis. | Dried Swietenia Senegalensis trunk bark powder is diluted at the rate of one teaspoonful in a teacup of lukewarm water and drunk as coffee twice a day (morning and evening). The same powder can be diluted in an alcoholic drink. Drink half a glass of liqueur once a day for at least 7 days. | No agreement |

Despite its ethnic character, the resources of traditional medicine remain the same from north to south. From Kinta to Nikki, via Kétou and Savè, the plants used by traditional practitioners to treat illnesses are identical.

However, due to cultural diversity, treatment rituals vary from one community to another. Traditional practitioners from Kinta, a Fon-speaking community, tend to believe that the strength of the treatments they offer patients comes from Vodoun (their traditional religion).

In contrast, their Nago counterparts from Kétou and Savè, and the Bariba from Nikki, have therapeutic practices that highlight the therapeutic virtues of plants. This differs from the occult practice of traditional medicine. For example, a traditional practitioner from Kaboua told us during our survey: "Traditional medicine is the plant, not the fetish".

What's more, the same remedy can be used for several different pathologies. This is one of the distinctive features of traditional medicine. The plant contains several active ingredients that are effective in treating a number of pathologies.

As a result, the plants used for treatment differ from one community to another.

# CHAPTER 4: FOUNDATIONS AND TECHNICAL BASES FOR THE PRACTICE OF TRADITIONAL MEDICINE

## A- Sociocultural and religious foundations

### 1- Socio-cultural constraints

According to a popular saying, "misfortune never comes on its own". The patient is psychologically and socially prepared to accept a supernatural cause for his illness. Research has revealed that socio-cultural, anthropological and religious considerations are the essential foundations of traditional medicine.

Unlike modern medicine, which is based on scientific and technical standards, the practices of Traditional Medicine draw their explanation and manifestation from the traditions of communities, religious practices, the culture of peoples and the anthropological realities of the social environment.

The tradipratician uses the material and spiritual means available to him and in his environment to heal, protect and maintain his psychological and physiological balance.

These sociological considerations are based on the supranatural and occult aspects of the cause of the illness. The healer will take all these aspects into account in his diagnosis. In contrast to allopathic medicine, which is based on an etiology derived from a semiological study of the patient and visible or measurable physical signs, traditional medicine, after taking an anamnesis, bases its diagnosis on cultural, religious or occult phenomena that are unverifiable and inaccessible to the uninitiated.

In such cases, the services of Fâ priests are called upon, and the resulting treatments are sometimes based on rituals involving offerings and prayers, depending on the case and the religious obedience. It's in these cases that the healing words replace plant, animal or mineral preparations and take the place of medicine.

In Kinta, when asked about the role of the priest of the fâ (bokonon in Fon) in traditional medicine, the answer was: "What is the role of the priest of the fâ in traditional medicine?

A tradipratician we spoke to replied as follows: "The bokonon plays an important role in the treatment of illnesses; it is he who helps us to know the origins of the illness".

The same tradipratician gives three origins of the disease:

- Illness can result from the anger of the gods to punish man's disobedience on earth. For example, disrespect for traditions can attract the wrath of the gods of earth, water, iron, forest etc. ;
- Illness can result from vengeance or simple malice (jealousy). It can result in poisoning or bewitchment;

- Finally, it can result from the displeasure of a dead relative offended by omission or neglect. In Africa, "the dead are not dead".

For example, in some circles, refusing to organize annual libations can be an offence to the dead and a way of attracting the "wrath of the dead".

Answering the same question about the role of Fâ in traditional medicine, another traditional practitioner in Kaboua said: "Thanks to IFA, we now know the names of the illnesses that disrupt man's organs and his life in general, as well as what can harm his health and temporal existence. Thanks to this knowledge, our parents were able to control diseases in one way or another in their time.

To understand the different answers to the question, the fâ is used to diagnose illnesses in Traditional Medicine.

In Kétou, a traditional practitioner explains liver disorders as a manifestation of the anger of "mothers". In the Yoruba anthropology of Nigeria and Benin, the term "mother" designates women who have the power of witchcraft.

As a remedy, the tradipratician indicates that the sick person must clean his body with a hen, asking the mothers to feel sorry for him and rid him of his illness. The hen is then immolated and cut into small pieces, immersed in red oil, placed in a calabash with other ingredients and taken to a crossroads (ori- iya-na -mèta) late at night.

### 2- Religious considerations

In the Kinta localities, the reference to Vodoun, the local traditional religion, as the sole holder of the power to heal is more accentuated, and the expression used by the traditional practitioner of religious obedience to affirm the healing power of the divinities is as follows:

"Vodoun nan go allo nu mi" which means, "the vodoun god will help us".

These are the fetishists who hold traditional therapeutic knowledge. Even when they use plant organs in their treatments, they deliberately attribute the healing power to their fetish rather than to the plants' therapeutic virtues.

For this category of traditional practitioners, traditional medicine is confused with religion.

This category of traditional healers is also to be found in all localities, using religion to propose solutions to health problems. For this latter category of healer, "Jesus Christ or Allah alone holds the power to heal".

Unfortunately, in the course of our surveys, we did not include this category of spiritual healing by traditional healers in our samples.

## B- Technical bases for the practice of Traditional Medicine

## 1- The tradipratician's long experience

The practice of traditional medicine is based on the tradipratician's long experience.

Indeed, the tradipratician has acquired mastery of the symptoms of certain illnesses through long experience in the practice of his art. To diagnose illness, his intelligence is the only source of inspiration.

When asked about the methods used to diagnose their patients' ailments, based on the descriptions given by the various traditional practitioners surveyed, and cross-checked by a state-qualified nurse, we were able to identify diagnostic methods, some of which, according to the health worker, are still used in modern medicine. These are :

- **Inspection.** With this method, the tradipratician observes the patient's expression, mine, lingual coating and physical appearance;
- **perception**. The tradipratician listens to the subject's voice, sniffing out his or her body odor;
- **questioning**. The tradipratician seeks to understand the patient's condition in order to make a more accurate diagnosis. He also asks about the course of the illness;
- **Palpation**. In other cases, he palpates the patient's arm to take his pulse, so as to know the strength, cadence and speed of his heartbeat. Sometimes, the whole body is palpated;
- **Percussion**. The tradipratician also uses this method, which involves tapping a part of the patient's body. This method is generally used when the patient is full of bloating. The belly is tapped with a single finger. The resonating sound differs according to whether the diagnosis is positive or negative.
- **auscultation.** With this method, the tradipratician looks for a small noise to ascertain whether the organ is active or not.
- **Taste.** To detect diabetes, for example, the tradipratician asks the patient to taste his or her own urine to assess the sugar content.
- It also uses the indicator flies or ants that invade the urine in case of sugar concentration.

## 2- Spiritual methods

To treat the diagnosed disease, the traditional practitioners surveyed use massage techniques with ointments based on plant or animal oils, scarification with powders obtained from fumigation, or spraying after drying plant, animal or mineral extracts.

They also use baths with solutions prepared as decoctions, macerations and/or infusions. These solutions can also be taken orally.

Sometimes, the leaves, bark or roots of plants are dried and made into incense. The smoke from this composition is supposed to destroy the evil forces haunting the patient.

The verb is sometimes used to accompany herbal preparations or animal and mineral extracts. It can also be used as a treatment in its own right.

To spiritually solicit the assistance of a sick person's dead relative, the traditional practitioner may prescribe offerings or sacrifices to be made as part of the treatment.

This is the case when the illness is of supernatural origin, i.e. when it is caused by evil forces. Rituals are also prescribed to combat these evil forces.

Finally, it should be pointed out that in the preparation of certain medicines, the tradipratician observes certain rituals and prohibitions that end up becoming totems for the patient.

In Kaboua, we were shown a remedy (a sauce) to treat infertility in women. The ingredients used to prepare the medicine must be crushed by a young girl who is still a long way from puberty. The disease has different meanings in traditional and modern medicine.

In Kétou, another traditional practitioner, whom we asked about a remedy used to treat hepatitis disorders, told us about the following ritual that accompanies his remedy:

He recommended the immolation of a hen after passing it over the body of the sick person; the hen would then be placed in a calabash at a crossroads. He explains this ritual by the fact that: "this illness is often caused by mothers; the sacrifice would serve to ask for their clemency and beg them to authorize the treatment of the illness with this remedy".

In Nago circles, the mother etymology refers to a woman initiated into the mystical power of witchcraft. In some African societies, women are presumed to possess witchcraft. They are therefore capable of causing illness in human beings. This is a matter of mystery in African culture. Any scientific explanation would risk being erroneous.

That's why in these societies, women of a certain age are both feared and revered.

Still based on cultural considerations, the only people capable of limiting the supremacy of women in society are traditional practitioners, some of whom derive their strength from the spirits to whom they devote all their beliefs through traditional religions.

In reality, the socio-cultural determinants that interfere with health and environmental issues relate to the socio-cultural characteristics of populations, their geographical distribution, their way of life and work, and their religious practices.

This is why the study was able to report that traditional medicine practices are based solely on the long experience of traditional practitioners handed down from generation to generation.

We also looked at the safety of the treatments offered by traditional healers, and the framework for collaboration between those involved in the two types of medicine.

# <u>CHAPTER 5</u>: SAFETY OF MEDICINES USED BY TRADITIONAL HEALERS AND FRAMEWORK FOR COLLABORATION BETWEEN TRADITIONAL HEALERS AND HEALTH WORKERS

## A- Safety of medicines used by traditional healers to treat illnesses

The safety of traditional medicines is a question of efficacy, safety and quality.

### 1- The therapeutic efficacy of traditional medicines used by traditional practitioners

Under the direction of Dr. GBAGUIDI Fernard from the Pharmacopoeia Study and Experimentation Laboratory, a specialized unit of the Beninese Center for Scientific and Technological Research (CBRST), biological tests were carried out on samples taken from medicinal plants used by traditional practitioners to treat illnesses.

The purpose of these tests is to carry out phytochemical screening and analyze the toxicity of these plants.

### a) ***<u>PHYTOCHEMICAL SCREENING</u>*** *:*

- **<u>Materials and methods</u>**

*Phytochemical screening was carried out using the P.J.Houjhton method based on staining and precipitation reactions.*

- *Alkaloids were characterized using Mayer's reagent (potassium iodomercurate reagent);*
- *Catechins and gallic tannins were determined using Stiasny's reagent;*
- *The cyanidine reaction (Shinoda reagent) was used to test flavonoids;*
- *The Liebermann-Buchard reaction was used to identify steroids and triterpenoids;*
- *The reaction with ferric chloride (FeCl3) was used to characterize the polyphenols;*
- *Saponosides were detected by measuring the foam height;*
- *The Born-Trager reaction was used to identify quinone derivatives;*

*The Guignard reaction was used to test cyanogenic derivatives.*

*The methods used in this analysis are summarized in the following table:*

| ***Active ingredient classes*** | ***Specific reagent and reactions*** |
|---|---|
| *Alkaloids* | *-Dragendorff (potassium iodobismuthate) ^ orange precipitate*<br>*-Mayer (potassium iodomercurate) ^ yellowish precipitate* |
| ***Tannins*** | *-FeCl3 ^ dark blue coloration* |
| ***Flavonoids*** | *Shinoda (cyanidine reaction) ^ orange-red coloration* |
| ***Anthocyanins*** | *-Red coloration in acid medium and purplish blue in alkaline medium* |
| ***Leucoanthocyanes*** | *-Hydrochloric alcohol (EtOH 50°/HClcc 2:1) ^ cherry red coloration* |
| ***Quinonic derivatives*** | *-Borntrager (reaction between quinonic rings in the medium NH4OH)*<br>*^ purplish red color* |
| ***Saponosides*** | *-Determination of foam index (positive if IM>100)* |
| ***Steroids and Terpenes*** | *-Liebermann-Burchard (Acetic anhydride-H2SO4cc 50:1)*<br>*^ violet coloring*<br>*-Kedde (dinitrobenzoic acid 1% in EtOH + NaOH 1N 1:1)*<br>*^ purple-red coloring (cardenolides)* |
| ***Cyanogenetic derivatives*** | *-Guignard (Paper impregnated with picric acid) ^ brown coloration* |
| | |
| ***Mucilage*** | *-Study the viscosity of infused and decocted products* |
| ***Essential oils*** | *-Steam drive*<br>*-Smell* |

## b) Results

***Product name: BRIDELIA FERRUGINEA LEAVES***

***Characteristics:*** *Powder* ***- Coffee***

***Therapeutic indications: Antidiabetic***

| *RESEARCH CHEMICAL GROUPS* | *RESULTS* |
|---|---|
| *ALKALOIDS* | + |
| *GALLIC TANNINS* | - |
| *CATECHIC TANNINS* | - |
| *FLAVONOIDS* | - |
| *ANTHOCYANES* | - |
| *LEUCOANTHOCYANES* | ++ |
| *QUINONE DERIVATIVES* | - |
| *SAPONOSIDES* | - |
| *STEROIDS*<br>*TRITERPENES* | -<br>+ |
| *MUCILAGE* | ++ |
| *REDUCING COMPOUNDS* | ++ |
| *CYANOGEN DERIVATIVES RESEARCH* | - |
| *FREE ANTHRACENE DERIVATIVES* | - |
| *COMBINEDANTRACEMIC DERIVATIVES: O-HETEROSIDES*<br>*C-HETEROSIDES* | -<br>- |
| *COUMARINES* | - |
| *CARDIOTONIC HETEROSIDES* | - |

*N.B: + : Present ; - : Absent ; ++: Present in large quantities*

***Product name : SOLANUM whole plant macerate LYCOPERSICUM MILL***

***Characteristics: Liquid - Light green Therapeutic indications: Antidiabetic,***

***antihypertensive, antimycotic, insecticide and anti-inflammatory.***

| *RESEARCH CHEMICAL GROUPS* | *RESULTS* |
|---|---|
| *ALKALOIDS* | + |
| *GALLIC TANNINS* | - |
| *CATECHIC TANNINS* | + |
| *FLAVONOIDS* | - |
| *ANTHOCYANES* | - |
| *LEUCOANTHOCYANES* | - |
| *QUINONE DERIVATIVES* | - |
| *SAPONOSIDES* | - |
| *STEROIDS* | - |
| *TRITERPENES* | ++ |
| *MUCILAGE* | + |
| *REDUCING COMPOUNDS* | - |
| *CYANOGEN DERIVATIVES RESEARCH* | - |
| *FREE ANTHRACENE DERIVATIVES* | - |
| *COMBINEDANTRACEMIC DERIVATIVES: O-HETEROSIDES* | - |
| *C-HETEROSIDES* | - |
| *COUMARINES* | + |
| *CARDIOTONIC HETEROSIDES* | - |

*N.B: + : Present ; - : Absent ; ++: Present in large quantities*

***Product name : LEAVES AND ROOTS OF* CYMBOPOGON Citratus *(DC) STAP***

***Characteristics: Powder - Coffee***

***Therapeutic indications: Antidiabetic***

| *RESEARCH CHEMICAL GROUPS* | *RESULTS* |
|---|---|
| *ALKALOIDS* | ++ |
| *GALLIC TANNINS* | - |
| *CATECHIC TANNINS* | - |
| *FLAVONOIDS* | - |
| *ANTHOCYANES* | - |

| | |
|---|---|
| *LEUCOANTHOCYANES* | - |
| *QUINONE DERIVATIVES* | - |
| *SAPONOSIDES* | - |
| *STEROIDS*<br>*TRITERPENES* | +<br>+ |
| *MUCILAGE* | ++ |
| *REDUCING COMPOUNDS* | ++ |
| *CYANOGEN DERIVATIVES RESEARCH* | - |
| *FREE ANTHRACENE DERIVATIVES* | - |
| *COMBINEDANTRACEMIC DERIVATIVES: O-HETEROSIDES*<br>*C-HETEROSIDES* | - - |
| *COUMARINES* | + |
| *CARDIOTONIC HETEROSIDES* | - |

*N.B: + : Present ; - : Absent ; ++: Present in large quantities*

***Product name :*** **CASSIA Alata LINN** ***Characteristics: Flower powder - Coffee Therapeutic indications: Anti-malarial***

| ***RESEARCH CHEMICAL GROUPS*** | ***RESULTS*** |
|---|---|
| *ALKALOIDS* | ++ |
| *GALLIC TANNINS* | - |
| *CATECHIC TANNINS* | - |
| *FLAVONOIDS* | ++ |
| *ANTHOCYANES* | ++ |
| *LEUCOANTHOCYANES* | - |
| *QUINONE DERIVATIVES* | + ***(pink)*** |
| *SAPONOSIDES* | - |
| *STEROIDS*<br>*TRITERPENES* | -<br>+ |
| *MUCILAGE* | ++ |
| *REDUCING COMPOUNDS* | ++ |
| *CYANOGEN DERIVATIVES RESEARCH* | - |

| *FREE ANTHRACENE DERIVATIVES* | - |
|---|---|
| *COMBINEDANTRACEMIC DERIVATIVES: O-HETEROSIDES*<br><br>*C-HETEROSIDES* | -<br>- |
| *COUMARINES* | ++ |
| *CARDIOTONIC HETEROSIDES* | - |

*__N.B:__ + : Present ; - : Absent ; ++: Present in large quantities*

***Product name HOLARHENA AFRICANA G. Don RABBETS, LEAVES, SCARKS, ROOTS, TRUNKS AND STALKS***

## *Characteristics: Powder - Coffee*

## *Therapeutic indications: Antidiabetics*

| ***RESEARCH CHEMICAL GROUPS*** | ***RESULTS*** |
|---|---|
| *ALKALOIDS* | - |
| *GALLIC TANNINS* | - |
| *CATECHIC TANNINS* | + |
| *FLAVONOIDS* | ++ |
| *ANTHOCYANES* | - |
| *LEUCOANTHOCYANES* | - |
| *QUINONE DERIVATIVES* | *+ **(purplish red)*** |
| *SAPONOSIDES* | ++ |
| *STEROIDS*<br><br>*TRITERPENES* | -<br><br>+ |
| *MUCILAGE* | ++ |
| *REDUCING COMPOUNDS* | ++ |
| *CYANOGEN DERIVATIVES RESEARCH* | - |
| *FREE ANTHRACENE DERIVATIVES* | + |
| *COMBINEDANTRACEMIC DERIVATIVES: O-HETEROSIDES*<br><br>*C-HETEROSIDES* | -<br>- |
| *COUMARINES* | ++ |
| *CARDIOTONIC HETEROSIDES* | - |

*N.B: + : Present ; - : Absent ; ++: Present in large quantities*

***Product name: MANGIFERA INDICA LINN SEED AMENDMENT***

***Characteristics: Powder - White***

***Therapeutic indications: Vermufige***

| *RESEARCH CHEMICAL GROUPS* | *RESULTS* |
|---|---|
| *ALKALOIDS* | ++ |
| *GALLIC TANNINS* | ++ |
| *CATECHIC TANNINS* | - |
| *FLAVONOIDS* | - |
| *ANTHOCYANES* | ++ |
| *LEUCOANTHOCYANES* | - |
| *QUINONE DERIVATIVES* | + *(pink)* |
| *SAPONOSIDES* | - |
| *STEROIDS*<br>*TRITERPENES* | -<br>+ |
| *MUCILAGE* | ++ |
| *REDUCING COMPOUNDS* | ++ |
| *CYANOGEN DERIVATIVES RESEARCH* | - |
| *FREE ANTHRACENE DERIVATIVES* | - |
| *COMBINEDANTRACEMIC DERIVATIVES: O-HETEROSIDES*<br>*C-HETEROSIDES* | -<br>- |
| *COUMARINES* | ++ |
| *CARDIOTONIC HETEROSIDES* | - |

*N.B: + : Present ; - : Absent ; ++: Present in large quantities*

**BRIDELIA FERRUGINEA Benth**

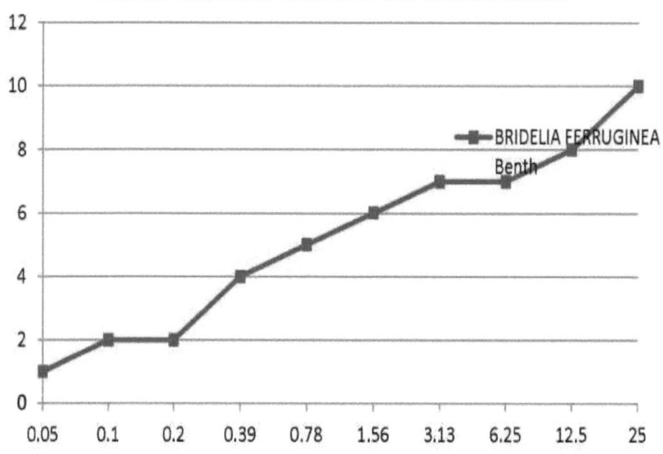


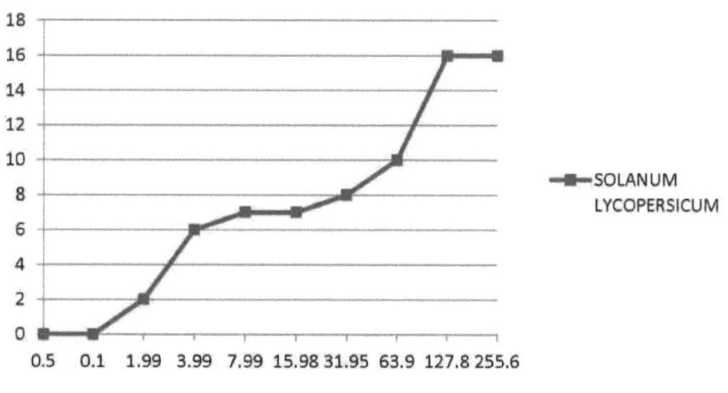


**SOLANUM LYCOPERSICUM**

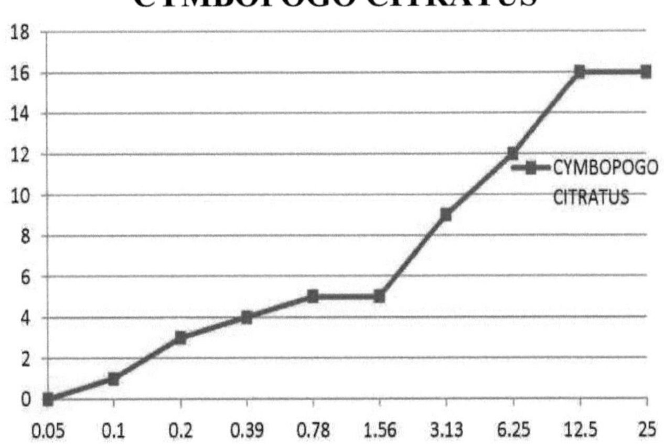
CYMBOPOGO CITRATUS
18
16
14
12
10
8
6
4
2
0
0.05
0.1
0.2
0.39
0.78
1.56
3.13
6.25
12.5
25
CYMBOPOGO CITRATUS

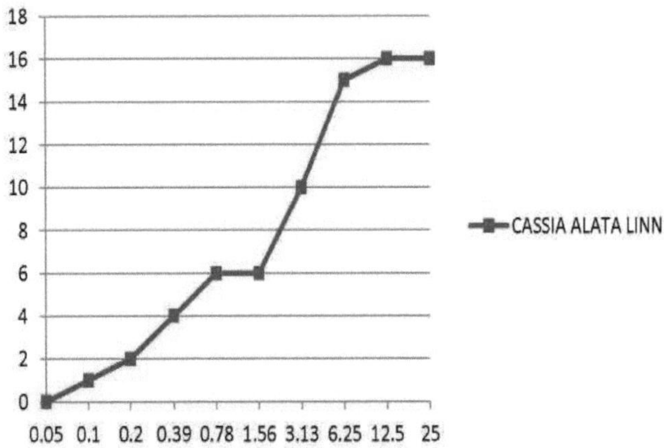
CASSIA ALATA LINN
18
16
14
12
10
8
6
4
2
0
0.05
0.1
0.2
0.39
0.78
1.56
3.13
6.25
12.5
25
CASSIA ALATA LINN

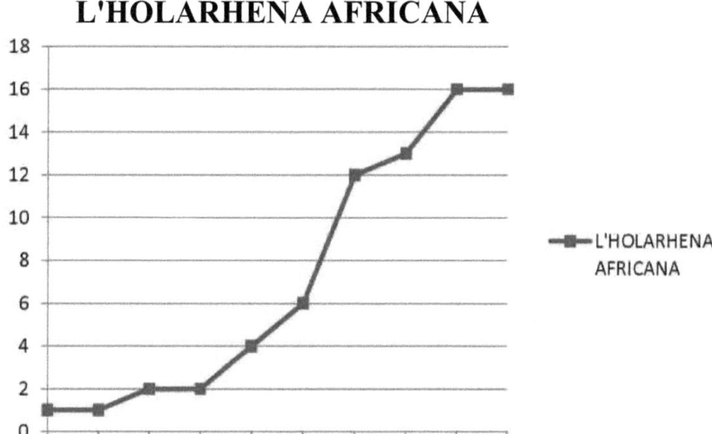
L'HOLARHENA AFRICANA
18
16
14
12
10
8
6
4
2
0
0.05 0.1 0.2 0.39 0.78 1.56 3.13 6.25 12.5 25
L'HOLARHENA AFRICANA

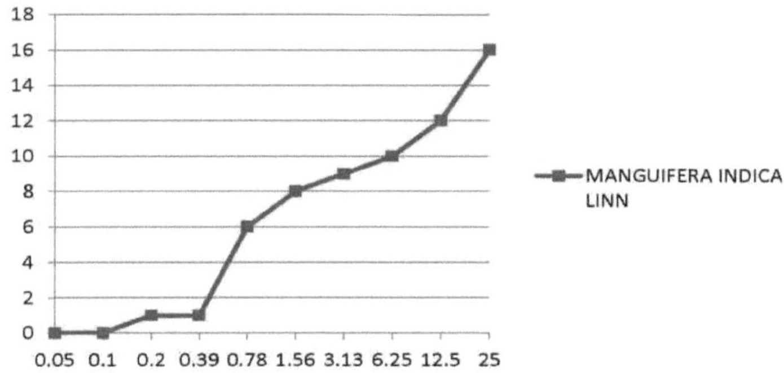
MANGUIFERA INDICA LINN
18
16
14
12
10
8
6
4
2
0
0.05 0.1 0.2 0.39 0.78 1.56 3.13 6.25 12.5 25
MANGUIFERA INDICA LINN

***Note:***

*Typical example of phytochemical screening interpretation*

## 1- Phytochemical analysis of "HÉMORROÏDOX BDK

**Results**

| *RESEARCH CHEMICAL GROUPS* | *RESULTS* |
|---|---|
| *ALKALOIDS* | +/- |
| *GALLIC TANNINS* | - |
| *CATECHIC TANNINS* | ++ |
| *FLAVONOIDS* | - |
| *ANTHOCYANES* | - |
| *LEUCOANTHOCYANES* | +++ |
| *QUINONE DERIVATIVES* | - |
| *SAPONOSIDES* | - |
| *STEROIDS*<br><br>*TRITERPENES* | +<br><br>- |
| *MUCILAGE* | ++ |
| *REDUCING COMPOUNDS* | ++ |
| *CYANOGEN DERIVATIVES RESEARCH* | - |
| *FREE ORGANIC DERIVATIVES* | - |
| *DERIVATIVESANTRACENICS COMBINES:*<br>*O-HETEROSIDES*<br><br>*C-HETEROSIDES* | - |
| *COUMARINES* | ++ |
| *CARDIOTONIC HETEROSIDES* | - |

***Results analysis***

*Analysis of phytochemical screening results shows the presence of catechic tannins, flavonoids, anthocyanins, leucoanthocyanins, reducing compounds, quinone derivatives, anthracene derivatives, mucilages, heterosides (cardiotonic), alkaloids and coumarins. The pharmacological properties of these major chemical groups : anthocyanins, leucoanthocyanins, reducing compounds (antioxidant activity, free radical scavenging, anti-inflammatory, anti-allergic, interaction with arachidonic acid metabolism, enzyme inhibitors), heterosides (broad spectrum of activity, depending on the genine), alkaloids (broad spectrum of biological activity), quinone derivatives (antibacterial, fungicidal,* ***antiparasitic****, laxative,* ***antitumoral,*** *urinary antiseptic, allergenic, etc.) may well account for the large number of compounds found in these plants.)* ***may well explain the therapeutic activity of these plants****.*

Time constraints have hampered our plans to extend this study to the clinical analysis of remedies obtained from these medicinal plants.

However, we can presume that the relief of patients in their suffering and even their satisfaction can serve as proof of the effectiveness of traditional remedies used in the management of disease.

Likewise, the tradipratician's long experience gives him confidence in the efficacy of his products.

The ineffectiveness of the remedy cannot be blamed on the traditional healer, because in our opinion he is not God.

Today, many synthetic drugs have been shown to be ineffective in the treatment of certain diseases and have been withdrawn from the market.

The safety of traditional medicines is one of the greatest challenges facing the policy of integrating traditional medicine into national healthcare systems. Traditional medicine still gives rise to strong reservations and skepticism about the benefits claimed by its practitioners.

**2- The safety of medicines used by traditional practitioners.**

Biological tests carried out at the pharmacognosy laboratory of the Beninese center for scientific and technological research on a number of medicinal plants collected in the field and used by traditional practitioners to treat illnesses have produced satisfactory results in terms of safety:

***Acute toxicity test***

***<u>Methods</u>***

*We worked with both sexes equally.*
*Initially, 06 concentrations of our extract were tested: 0.01mg/Kg, 0.1mg/kg, 1mg/kg, 10mg/kg, 100mg/kg, 1g/kg on 06 rats, with 01 rat for each concentration. Based on the observations made at the end of this first phase, a*

*second series of tests was carried out by preparing a series of 05 batches of rats: 1st batch: administration of the white control (DMSO in this case) 2nd batch: administration of an extract concentration for which we have 0% Mort*
*Batch 3: administration of an extract concentration of between 5 and 50% mortality*
*4th batch: administration of an extract concentration for which mortality is between 50 and 95%.*
*Batch 5: administration of an extract concentration for which 100% is obtained mortality*
*Based on the dose-response curve obtained, the LD50, LD5, LD95*
*Tests are validated if LD50/DL5= LD95/DL50*
*And if DL95/DL5: Safety Index (SI)*
*If IS >10: very good extract*
*5<IS<10: extract to be used with caution*
*IS< 5: toxic extract, be very careful*

*These extracts were administered by gavage (per os) in a maximum volume of 5ml. Observations on animals are made over a period of one week (or more than 15 days for the acute toxicities we observe).*

### *Note on larval toxicity*

*To assess toxicity on the basis of IC50 values, we have followed the correspondence table (table n ) drawn up by* ***Mireille Mousseux in 1995.***

*Table n: Correspondence between IC50 and toxicity*

| *IC50* | *Toxicity* |
|---|---|
| *IC50>100 g-giml or 0.1mg/mL* | - |
| *11)1)ugmLIC5i0>51)ug mL or 0.1mg/mL> IC50>0.050mg/mL* | + |
| *50LigmLI(gı g1))LigmL or 0.050mg/mL> IC50>0.01mg/mL* | + + |
| *ICgi 10ugmL or 0.01mg/mL* | + + + |

***Acute toxicity assessment - BRIDELIA FERRUGINEA***

| ***For medu product*** | ***Administered dose*** | ***Method of administration*** | ***Comments*** |
|---|---|---|---|
| | | | |

| | | | |
|---|---|---|---|
| *Hot water extract*<br><br>*(med. traditional)*<br><br>*Purpose: assessment of acute toxicity* | ***400 mg powder/kg/day*** | ***Feeding***<br><br>*(distilled water)* | • *No change in urine output*<br>• *No influence on weight gain*<br>• *No liver or kidney damage*<br>• ***Stained urine after two days of treatment*** |

## - *SOLANUM LYCOPERSICUM MILL*

| ***For medu product*** | ***Administered dose*** | ***Method of administration*** | ***Comments*** |
|---|---|---|---|
| *Aqueous liquid*<br><br>*(traditional med.)*<br><br>*Purpose: assessment of acute toxicity* | ***300 mg liquid/kg/day*** | ***Feeding***<br><br>*(distilled water)* | • *No change in urine output*<br>• *No influence on weight gain*<br>• *No liver or kidney damage*<br>• ***Stained urine after two days of treatment*** |

## - CYMBOPOGON Citratus *(DC) STAP*

| ***For medu product*** | ***Administered dose*** | ***Method of administration*** | ***Comments*** |
|---|---|---|---|
| *Hot water extract*<br><br>*(traditional med)*<br><br>*Purpose: assessment of acute toxicity* | ***400 mg powder/kg/day*** | ***Feeding***<br><br>*(distilled water)* | • *No change in urine output*<br>• *No influence on weight gain*<br>• *No liver or kidney damage*<br>• ***Stained urine after two days of treatment*** |

## - *CASSIA ALATA LINN*

| ***For medu product*** | ***Administered dose*** | ***Method of administration*** | ***Comments*** |
| --- | --- | --- | --- |
| *Hot water extract*<br>*(traditional med.)*<br><br>*Purpose: assessment of acute toxicity* | ***400 mg powder/kg/day*** | ***Feeding***<br>*(distilled water)* | • *No change in urine output*<br>• *No influence on weight gain*<br>• *No liver or kidney damage*<br>- |

***- HOLARHENA AFRICANA G. RODS, LEAVES, ECOCREES, ROOTS, TRUNKS AND STALKS***

| ***For medu product*** | ***Administered dose*** | ***Method of administration*** | ***Comments*** |
| --- | --- | --- | --- |
| *Hot water extract*<br>*(traditional med.)*<br><br>*Purpose: assessment of acute toxicity* | ***400 mg powder/kg/day*** | ***Feeding***<br>*(distilled water)* | • *No change in urine output*<br>• *No influence on weight gain*<br>• *No liver or kidney damage*<br>• ***Decreased motricity at doses higher than 450 mg powder/kg/day*** |

***- FINE MANGIFERA INDICA LINN KERNEL***

| ***For medu product*** | ***Administered dose*** | ***Method of administration*** | ***Comments*** |
| --- | --- | --- | --- |

| *Hot water extract*<br><br>*(traditional med.)*<br><br><br><br><br>*Purpose: assessment of acute toxicity* | ***300 mg powder/kg/day*** | ***Feeding***<br><br>*(distilled water)* | • *No change in urine output*<br>• *No influence on weight gain*<br>• *No liver or kidney damage*<br>• ***Decreased motricity at doses higher than 350 mg powder/kg/day*** |
|---|---|---|---|

## 1- Pharmaceutical quality of remedies used by traditional practitioners.

On the basis of the results and observations made in the field, the pharmaceutical quality of the traditional medicines used shows qualitative shortcomings:

- Packaging still needs improvement. The diseases treated with the remedy are barely legible on a piece of paper or sometimes cardboard, or even a piece of cement paper;
- The tradipratician did not write the dosage, contraindications, chemical composition or expiration date on the packaging.

## B- Framework for collaboration between traditional healers and health workers

There is often a lack of trust between traditional healers and modern medical practitioners. In the eyes of the latter, health workers are the colonizer's henchmen, and health facilities are mere relays for the colonial administration.

During colonial times, traditional practitioners were persecuted and driven underground. Despite acts of recognition of traditional medicine by national governments as well as by international and regional bodies, the idea of rejecting traditional medicine has not changed.

traditional medicine has always haunted traditional practitioners, most of whom are illiterate.

Traditional practitioners and health workers don't trust each other. The former see the latter as spies for Western laboratories. Health workers, for their part, have a complex about the superiority that scientific and technological progress confers on them.

The latter hide behind standards to systematically reject all other approaches that deviate from them.

In health centers, traditional remedies are systematically banned from use, on the pretext that they suffer from a lack of proof of efficacy, safety and quality.

In the health facilities surveyed, no traditional health care is available, and health workers refuse to prescribe it to patients.

On the whole, health workers in the health facilities surveyed have very little knowledge of traditional therapeutic methods.

96% of the agents surveyed said they had no knowledge of traditional medicine.

Similarly, 92% said they did not collaborate with traditional practitioners in the practice of their profession.

On the other hand, 02% of these agents admitted to having been treated once themselves by a traditional practitioner.

# PART THREE: DISCUSSION

## CHAPTER 6: ANALYSIS OF RESULTS

### A- Analysis

#### 1- Socio-cultural and religious foundations of Traditional Medicine

Over 2,000 years old, traditional Chinese medicine has been able to free itself from socio-cultural constraints and religious beliefs and become universal. It makes abundant use of advances in science and technology, notably biomedical technologies. The Chinese practitioner of traditional medicine uses modern diagnostic methods before prescribing treatments.

Acupuncture is a hallmark of Chinese medicine that has already been used around the world.

How else are we to understand that cultural and religious foundations sometimes lead to unhealthy practices in traditional medicine, aggravating the patient's already fragile state of health despite the guarantee of harmlessness resulting from years of use of the same remedy?

Confusion between traditional medicine and certain traditional religious practices could compromise the evolution of traditional medicine alongside modern medicine.

Every people has its own wonderful legends about traditional medicine. In Africa, the history of traditional medicine is linked to the brilliant civilization of the continent's first communities.

More than three centuries later, traditional medicine can still claim to be part of the cultural heritage of the different communities that populate Africa.

#### 2- Practical basics of Traditional Medicine

Like all science, modern medicine is progressing, while certain diagnostic methods used in traditional medicine remain unchanged.

For example, instead of using urine on a white cloth to diagnose yellow fever in traditional medicine, modern medicine now uses reagents for color comparison, as well as qualitative and quantitative analysis of bilirubin content.

Diagnostic results are obtained according to the color change of the reagent papers.

However, new tools are increasingly being used in medicine. Technological advances now make it possible to diagnose with much greater precision.

The treatments administered are the result of lengthy scientific studies that ensure the efficacy, dose safety and quality of the drugs prescribed.

However, patients treated in conventional health facilities are confronted with a number of constraints, not the least of which are the following:

- The patient is not treated as a whole; in fact, the modern doctor only deals with pathological complaints. The patient's social and psychological problems are often ignored;
- The cost of treatment is one of the main reasons why the majority of poor people do not have access to formal healthcare.
- Disparities in the distribution of healthcare personnel, infrastructure and equipment are just some of the shortcomings that still plague modern medicine, and are the main reasons why people choose traditional medicine.

In rural communities, living conditions are still precarious in some places due to poverty.

As a result of numerous experiments, these communities have come to know a number of plants for curing snakebites. Now, if you've been bitten by a snake, you know which plants to use.

As far as diagnostic methods are concerned, modern medicine makes good use of modern technologies to achieve fast and accurate results, while traditional medicine still leaves the therapist uncertain.

However, traditional medicine has nothing to worry about, even if it is important to note that the option of integrating traditional medicine into the official health care system is based on the premise that practices relating to Traditional Medicine should be included alongside those already conventionalized and linked to biomedical medicine.

**3- Disease management remedies**

The problem of traditional medicines in Benin is one of quality and availability. To achieve the objective of integration, it is necessary to ensure the quantitative and qualitative production of traditional medicines for the treatment of diseases.

**a) Quantitative production**

The quantitative production of traditional medicines depends first and foremost on the availability of raw materials (particularly plant materials).

Natural flora as the sole source of medicinal plants will not ensure the sustainability of traditional medicine in Benin.

One of the weaknesses of the national pharmacopoeia and traditional medicine program is its failure to effectively implement the program to promote medicinal plant gardens in Benin.

The few gardens that have survived the bad weather and lack of maintenance have become, for the most part, the exclusive property of the presidents of the local structures of the national association of traditional medicine practitioners in Benin (ANAPRAMETRAB).

The development of botanical gardens is becoming one of the priorities of the policy to integrate traditional medicine into the national health system.

The small gardens planted here and there, usually in the backyards of traditional practitioners' homes, cannot meet the constant and growing needs of industrial production of traditional medicines.

The integration of traditional medicine provides an opportunity to promote a new agricultural sector: the cultivation of medicinal plants. This new sector opens up entrepreneurial prospects, creating numerous jobs and wealth to boost the country's economic growth.

In terms of health, the importance of traditional medicine is well established. However, if traditional medicines are to be available in quantity, plant species must be protected and safeguarded, hence the relevance of the expression: **"Save the plants that save lives".**

**b) Qualitative production**

The effects of traditional medicines depend on where they are grown, when they are harvested and how they are prepared.

Some substances need to be dried in the sun and others out of it; some need to be turned into pills and others into powder; some need to be boiled in water and others macerated or toasted with alcohol.

Furthermore, to ensure a regular and sustainable supply of improved traditional medicines, it is essential to create the conditions for quantitative and standardized production. This will undoubtedly require the promotion of a local traditional medicine production industry.

Despite the richness of Benin's natural flora in medicinal plants, the country has very few industrial units producing safe traditional medicines.

Many initiatives in this field have run out of steam and faded away. The scientific research that must precede the production of improved traditional medicines has lacked funding.

No biological or clinical tests could be carried out on the traditional remedies used by the traditional practitioners surveyed for this study.

At this stage of our research, no scientific evidence is available to support the therapeutic efficacy and dose-related safety of the remedies listed. The study will undoubtedly be continued.

**Nevertheless, "Even if it clashes with the principles of modern, conventional science, traditional medicine today presents itself as the African solution to the**

**challenges of health and development" (WHO, 2005).**

In many developed countries, the popularity of herbal medicine has been boosted by concerns about the harmful effects of chemical drugs, by the questioning of allopathic approaches and presumptions, and by the general public's increasingly easy access to health information.

Increased life expectancy has multiplied the risk of developing debilitating chronic diseases such as cardiovascular disease, diabetes, mental disorders, HIV/AIDS and tuberculosis.

For many patients, herbal medicines seem to offer a less aggressive way of managing these types of illnesses than allopathy.

The over-the-counter (OTC) herbal remedies industry has suffered a setback over the past three years, mainly due to bad press caused by quality issues.

However, there are many indications that the demand for herbal medicines is increasing. These include :

- dissatisfaction with Western medicine;
- rising healthcare costs;
- cultural, spiritual and religious aspirations;
- interest in a return to a more natural way of life;
- the public's growing desire to take control of their own health;
- and increased recognition of the therapeutic value of food.

**Appreciation of the high use of Traditional Medicine worldwide, in Africa and in Benin**

In 2002, according to World Health Organization statistics, the use of traditional medicine was as follows:

**- In the West**

- 48% in Australia;
- 70% in Canada;
- 42% in the United States;
- 38% in Belgium;
- 75% in France.

**- In Africa**

- 70% in Sudan ;
- 30% in Uganda;

- 60% in Mali and Ghana;
- 80% in Benin.

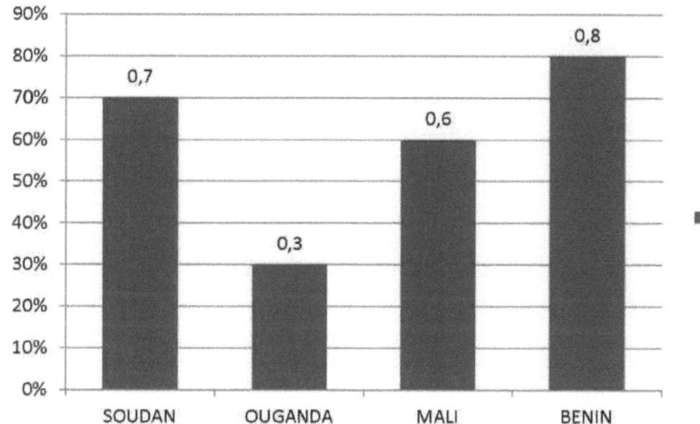


**Figure 1**: Graphical representation

Growing medicinal plants involves a number of risks:

- The international plant market ;
- Standards on good agricultural practices and good harvesting practices for medicinal plants; , marketing and regulations.

However, markets remain uncertain: they can disappear suddenly if the plant is deemed unsafe for consumption, and they are subject to fluctuations in demand.

**4- Collaboration between practitioners from the two medical orders**

In practice, health-care workers who are highly attached to medical standards find it difficult to accept the approach and ethics of traditional medicine.

As for traditional practitioners, they are rightly or wrongly suspicious of their collaboration with health workers.

However, it is important to recognize that there is now a willingness on both sides to work together. What remains to be done is to define the framework and form of this collaboration.

However, we believe that at the current stage of knowledge of traditional medicine within communities, any policy should aim to keep the traditional practitioner in the community, where he or she contributes to access to primary health care within the limits of his or her knowledge.

Under these conditions, the status that best suits the tradipratician's situation is that of self-employed worker, which does not exclude the possibility of collaboration with modern doctors, but at least avoids placing the tradipratician under tutelage.

They are not motivated by the collaboration framework that turns traditional practitioners into mere auxiliaries of the health administration, without any compensation.

Traditional medicine should develop separately, but of course it needs to be supported by appropriate legislation. Traditional medicine needs a methodological update.

It also needs appropriate technologies for the identification, production and development of traditional remedies to increase their medical, economic and socio-cultural benefits and acceptance.

The lack of collaboration is not just between traditional practitioners and health workers!

Traditional practitioners are not aware of the institutions responsible for overseeing the traditional medicine sub-sector.

With the national pharmacopoeia and traditional medicine program, the institution in charge of drawing up and implementing the national policy for integrating traditional medicine, we need to improve our collaborative approach with all traditional medicine players throughout the country.

The official recognition of ANAPRAMETRAB as the sole organization by decree in 1986 gave it legitimacy and representativeness that had not been compromised until then.

The program must work to unite all the players in traditional medicine within this melting pot. Unfortunately, this is not yet the case.

It's a minority of traditional practitioners, mostly in the south of the country, who are busy taking advantage of the seminars and workshops in which they are always the only participants. Insufficient financial resources should not be used as a pretext for concentrating the program's activities in one part of the country.

In the field, 93% of the traditional practitioners we met had never taken part in any of the program's activities (forums, seminars and training workshops).

### B- Other ways of integrating traditional medicine

#### 1- Training for traditional practitioners

The training of traditional practitioners is an important part of the process of integrating traditional medicine into the official healthcare system. It is a point of collaboration between the two medical orders.

The scientific and technological advantage of modern medicine lies in its universality.

Benin lags far behind in the teaching of traditional medicine.

Even in the training programs of medical schools and faculties, no module is devoted to the teaching of traditional medicine, whereas in France, where conventional medicine is booming, a department of Traditional Medicine has been set up at the University of Bobigny.

So if Africans don't quickly become aware of their endogenous therapeutic heritage, the West will get hold of it again, like other raw materials, and sell it back to us at a very high price.

In contrast to the Chinese system, which boasts numerous institutes and schools for training in traditional medicine, Benin does not yet have any schools for training in traditional medicine.

To meet the training needs of traditional practitioners, the Programme National de la Pharmacopée et de la Médecine Traditionnelle

(PNPMT) organizes a series of training courses supported by teaching manuals. These include, for example :

- The training seminar for traditional practitioners on the management of uncomplicated malaria is supported by a protocol for the management of uncomplicated malaria.

  malaria based on effective traditional practices in Benin. This document was produced in 2009;

- Training in the management of STIs and HIV/AIDS in Benin, with a supporting training manual also produced in 2009;
- In January 2011, a training seminar was held on good practices in the fight against HIV/AIDS in traditional medicine in Benin, with documentation available:
- Also in January 2011, another training course, this time for healthcare professionals, supported by a manual introducing healthcare professionals to the systems of education and transmission of knowledge in traditional medicine in Benin.

The ideal would be to create a diploma course to welcome all those who wish to turn to this medicine and make it their profession.

**2- Protecting endogenous therapeutic knowledge and know-how**

Protecting endogenous knowledge remains a challenge in the policy of integrating traditional medicine into the official health system.

What's the point of improving other forms of integration if Africa's therapeutic heritage is being systematically pirated or even sold off?

Or what does the future hold for traditional medicine when Africa's natural flora is being plundered by Western powers?

These are just some of the questions that need to be answered in the process of integrating traditional medicine into the official healthcare system.

Through education, information and communication, we need to popularize legal texts and make it easier for people to access measures to protect endogenous knowledge.

# CHAPTER 7: REASONS FOR HOPE

The road to integrating traditional medicine into Benin's healthcare system is long and strewn with many pitfalls. But there is hope. There are three reasons for this hope:

- political will ;
- mobilization and advocacy actions;
- Raising people's collective awareness of Traditional Medicine.

**A- Political will**

**1- Mission of the national program for traditional pharmacopoeia and medicine**

This commitment led to the creation of a national pharmacopoeia and traditional medicine program in 1996. Placed under the supervision of the Ministry of Health, the program's mission is to :

- Development and implementation of a legal framework for the practice of traditional medicine and pharmacopoeia;
- The construction of traditional medicine care units in all departments;
- Technical capacity building for traditional medicine practitioners;
- Continuing to set up botanical gardens to ensure self-sufficiency in the supply of medicinal plants, which continue to depend on natural flora;
- Setting up a database on medicinal plants.

**2- Evaluation of program actions**

The gap between programming and implementation of the PNPMT is very wide. However, significant results have been achieved:

- A decree laying down the ethical principles and conditions of practice of traditional medicine and an interministerial order regulating advertising for traditional pharmacopoeia and medicine make up the bulk of the legal arsenal in the field of traditional medicine in Benin;
- The program has been more active in capacity building.

To this end, training manuals on the management of malaria, sexually transmitted diseases (STDs) and HIV/AIDS have been produced.

Literacy training for traditional practitioners, most of whom are illiterate, has not been very successful.

In the field of research, a research protocol to validate the efficacy of traditional medicines used in the treatment of malaria, and clinical tests to identify and validate traditional products effective in the treatment of malaria and HIV/AIDS.

### 8- Mobilization and advocacy actions

Integrating traditional medicine into the national health system is a development issue. Numerous mobilization and advocacy actions by national players and the international community are underway.

Every June 12, Benin commemorates the national day of traditional medicine. 2011 was no exception. Placed under the evocative theme: "Entrepreneurship at the service of the local industry producing medicines from medicinal plants", this year corresponds to the eleventh day. The day marks the awareness of the authorities in charge of Traditional Medicine of the economic stakes involved.

The day also marks the start of a partnership between the Ministry of Health (MS) and the Ministry of Industry, Trade and Small and Medium-sized Enterprises (MICPME).

This partnership testifies to the MICPME's interest in the traditional medicine sector as a means of improving the industrial fabric, promoting small and medium-sized enterprises (SMEs) and entrepreneurship in Benin.

## C- Collective awareness of the therapeutic and economic implications of traditional medicine

The massive adherence to traditional medicine is not just proof of the resignation of the majority of the more than 80% of the population who use this form of healthcare.

It may also be a strong signal of the population's awareness of the therapeutic importance of this medicine in the management of emerging diseases.

In fact, a constant and current body of literature testifies to the absence of side-effects in treatments based on herbal medicines. Even in affluent environments, where access to healthcare is not a financial concern, traditional therapeutic treatments are increasingly tolerated and in demand.

Traditional practitioners and other traditional medicine specialists are also aware that only improved traditional medicines (ITMs) can effectively contribute to improving access to primary healthcare.

Benin's health authorities have understood this, and are working tirelessly to develop regulations governing the production and marketing of improved traditional medicines.

To qualify as an improved traditional medicine in Benin, two conditions must currently be met:

- The drug must be accompanied by a certificate of analysis: Phytochemical Screening issued by an accredited pharmacognosy laboratory.

- A toxicity study certificate issued by an approved laboratory.

For the time being, the long experience of traditional practitioners in using their remedies to treat illnesses lends credence to proof of efficacy, pending the adoption of a standard protocol for research into the efficacy of traditional remedies used by traditional practitioners to treat illnesses.

The cost of bringing medicines into compliance is no longer a handicap for traditional practitioners, who increasingly understand the need to form multidisciplinary teams to produce improved traditional medicines in quantity and quality.

This strategy has had a positive impact on local production of traditional medicines from the national pharmacopoeia.

In conjunction with the 9ème Day of Traditional Medicine commemorated on August 30, 2011, the Association Nationale des Praticiens de la Médecine Traditionnelle du Bénin (ANAPRAMETRAB) organized the first edition of the national fair for improved traditional medicines.

Over forty traditional practitioners took part in this unique scientific and commercial event, offering the public a range of traditional remedies of high pharmaceutical quality.

All the remedies exhibited at this fair are the result of endogenous therapeutic knowledge submitted to the expertise of proven and accredited laboratories.

This event represents a milestone in the implementation of the policy of integrating traditional medicine into the Beninese health system.

**D- Scientific motivations**

Traditional therapeutic potential is increasingly being replaced by scientific motivations, leading to in-depth knowledge, rehabilitation and upgrading of the substratum of this ancestral art of healing, which still saves a significant proportion of our populations today.

Patients in rural and suburban areas, and even a considerable number of those in typically urban areas, now turn to traditional practitioners of medicine, where there is an ever-increasing number of traditional practitioners, as well as significant trafficking in processed materials and medicines.

From the moment when cultural achievements make it possible to relieve and definitively cure patients who trust endogenous knowledge in this specific field, and who devote themselves fully to it because of the convincing results obtained, there is a need for scientific and technological motivation;

At the same time, there is an obligation to pursue research into cultural, economic and social issues.

The main aim of this research is to safeguard the national heritage of knowledge in all areas related to health, the search for balance and harmony in populations, the social environment and ecosystems, and so on.

In addition, they aim for endogenous, self-centered and self-sustaining development by healthy populations and their permanent salvation in a naturally healthy and sanitized environment.

Traditional medicine is firmly rooted in the culture and traditions of communities. Its judicious use is an asset in achieving the goal of health for all through primary health care.

This is why harmonization and fruitful collaboration with modern medicine must be a political and legal option, with a few precautions:

- Creation of a multidisciplinary institute based on a sufficiently flexible system to secure access for traditional practitioners to public health services;
- Codification of the practice of the profession without alienation of any kind of the tradipratician;
- Introducing safe traditional medicines into everyday practice and developing reciprocal scientific and cultural enrichment.

These aspects are essential to the policy of integrating traditional medicine, and must be pursued with the requisite resources and realistic mechanisms in the interests of public health in Benin.

# GENERAL CONCLUSION AND SUGGESTIONS

In reality, based on the socio-cultural foundation of traditional medicine, the problem of promoting it in the official healthcare system does not arise in terms of its integration.

For reasons of efficiency, each medicine must remain in its own place, retaining its originality. Countries such as China and Vietnam have reconciled the two types of medicine without seeking to integrate them.

And if we are aware that traditional medicine derives most of its resources from plants, it becomes urgent to promote the cultivation of medicinal plants.

This promotion involves rolling out the policy of developing medicinal plant gardens in all Benin's communes.

In addition, to strengthen the development of traditional medicine, Benin needs an institute dedicated to research and training in traditional medicine and pharmacopoeia.

Such an institute needs to bring together a wide range of skills.

We also need to set up a communication and information network on the progress made in traditional medicine.

This study opens the way for further research into the remedies identified during the search.

# APPENDIX

## DATA COLLECTION TOOLS

### I- Interview guide for patients

**Question 1:** Why are you here?

**Answer:** I'm here because I'm sick.

**Question 2**: Are you from the village?

**Answer:** I'm local, my village is two kilometers from here.

**Question 3:** How did you hear about this traditional practitioner?

**Answer**: Our villages are close to each other, so we all know each other. We know who does what in each of our villages.

**Question 4**: How long have you been seeing a tradipratician?

**Answer: I** arrived at the tradipraticien NAGONOUTA two weeks later.

**Question n° 5 :** Have you ever consulted a health agent for your illness?

**Answer:** No, I did not consult a health agent before coming to the tradipratician.

**Question 6:** How has your state of health changed since you came to the tradipratician?

**Answer:** I thank God. I'm getting better and better.

**Question n°7:** What kind of medicines are you treated with? Specifically, are the remedies that the tradipratician administers to you in powder, solution, macerated or incantatory form?

**Answer:** A bit of everything

**Question 8:** Why did you choose to go to a traditional practitioner instead of a health center?

**Answer:** I don't have enough money to pay for the more expensive care at health centers.

**Question 9**: How much have your treatments cost since you first went to the tradipratician?

**Answer**: So far, I haven't paid anything to the tradipratician.

**Question 10: Does** your traditional practitioner treat you on credit?

**Answer**: Not on credit, but he hasn't taken anything from me since I moved in.

**Question n°11:** Perhaps he's waiting for you to recover before letting you know the cost of your treatment?

**Answer**: I don't know.

**Question 12:** Did you have a special relationship with this traditional practitioner?

**Answer**: Maybe

**Question n°13 :** Can you tell us how satisfied you are by entrusting your health care to a tradipratician?

**Answer**: The tradipratician gives us all the attention we need in all our complaints, and we feel right at home," adds another. "He's available day and night to respond to patients' requests.

**NB:** The interview was conducted with patients and carers. The answers given do not contradict each other.

## II- Group discussion guide for traditional practitioners

**Question 1**: How long have you been practicing traditional medicine?

**Answers**: I've been practicing traditional medicine for 10, 12, 16, 20, 22, 24, 26 and 30 years, according to the many people who took part in the interview.

**Question 2:** How did you get into the profession?

**Answers:** I inherited it from my father; my grandfather; my uncle. Only one participant replied that he had learned the practice from friends and then travelled to Nigeria to perfect his skills.

**Question 3**: What diseases do you treat?

**Answers**: A little of everything

**Question n°4:** How many patients do you receive per month and per year?

**Answer**: To receive or to treat, retorted a participant, who insisted on the nuance, adding that we don't receive all the patients we treat in our homes. There are urgent and prompt interventions that we carry out wherever we are called. He adds: "If it's treated, there are a lot of them, without being able to say how many.

**Question 5**: How much does it cost to care for your family?

**Answers**: It depends on the complication of the disease and also on the availability of the plant, animal or mineral materials used to prepare the remedies used to treat the disease.

**Question 6**: What about simple malaria?

**Answers:** One hundred to two hundred CFA francs at least to buy plants at the market if in an urban center. If you're in a rural area, you'll just have to send a child into the bush to get the plants you need, with no financial implications.

**Question 7**: Yet you are accused of offering care that is more expensive than that offered by health facilities.

**Answers:** False, all participants agreed. However, it's important to distinguish between the care offered in town and that offered in our villages, said one participant. In town, most of those who claim to be traditional healers without any experience are the ones who tarnish the image of traditional healers and sully the profession. A tradipratician is never rich, yet he's protected from the need for food, because his many benefits bring him rewards in the form of material and financial goods, and even immaterial goods such as a wife (the whole audience bursts into laughter).

**Question 8**: How do you recognize genuine traditional healers from fake ones?

**Answers**: In traditional society, each clan and family has its own role and is recognized as such. Thus, there are blacksmiths, who take care of instruments of war and agriculture; weavers, hunters; divinatory priests. It is among these last two communities that we find powerful healers. This heritage has been handed down from generation to generation. In our villages, it's easy to recognize each family's lineage and activities.

**Question 9**: What are the main materials you use in preparing your remedies?

**Answers**: We mainly use plants, animal and mineral extracts.

**Question 10**: What are your treatment methods?

**Answers**: Our treatments are either herbal (phytotherapy), and/or based on spiritual beliefs.

**Question n°** 11: Do you work with health facilities?

**Answers**: Not at all

**Question** 12: What are the reasons for this?

**Responses**: The framework doesn't lend itself to an environment characterized by mistrust between us and health workers.

**Question** n°13 : Are you ready to collaborate with these health workers?

**Answers**: We want to improve our performance.

**Question** n°14: What is your last resort if your treatment fails?

**Answers**: We refer patients to the nearest health center or return them to their homes.

**Question n°** 15: How do you plan to ensure the succession?

**Answers**: Our children will take over.

**Question n°16** Do you think that a training school in Traditional Medicine could contribute to the promotion of this alternative healthcare method?

**Answers** : Many

**Question** 17: Have you ever taken part in capacity-building training courses for traditional practitioners in Benin?

**Answers**: Not everyone

**Question n°18**: What role do incantatory words play in the effectiveness of traditional remedies?

**Answers**: The word magnifies plants and commands them to act in a healing way.

**Question n°19**: What are the threats to the survival of traditional medicine in Benin?

**Answers**: The precariousness of traditional medicine resources, particularly plant materials.

## III- QUESTIONNAIRE: FOR HEALTH AGENTS

NAME & SURNAME OF INVESTIGATOR :

INVESTIGATOR CODE :

DATE OF SURVEY :

DEPARTEMENT :

COMMUNE :

ARRONDISSEMENT

VILLAGE/NEIGHBORHOOD

How long have you been in the locality? .................. In Year

**1) Geographical area**:

/__/ Urban /__/ Suburban /__/ Rural

THE SURVEY:

Respondent number /__/ given by interviewer

Ethnicity to be ....... specified

Gender /__/ Male /__/ Female

AgeIn ............. year

**2) Education level**

/__/ Primary /__/ Secondary /__/ Higher education

**3) Marital status**

/__/ Married /__/ Single /__/ Divorced /__/ Widowed

**4) Residence status**

/__/ Owner /__/ Renter /__/ Free lodger

_ // .................................................. OthersSpecify

**5) Professional experience**

How long have you been in the profession?

_ // ........ MonthSpecify // ______YearSpecify

In the body?

/__/ 1 to 10 years /__/ 10 to 20 years /__/ More than 20 years.

**6) Epidemiological status**

What are the most common illnesses recorded in your consultations?

/__/ Malaria /__/ Hypertension

/__/ Diabetes /__/ Asthma /__/ Hepatitis

/__/ Sickle cell disease /__/ Diarrheal diseases

/__/ Female Sterility /__/ Sexual Impotence

/__/ HIV/AIDS

__// Other illnesses to be ............................... specified.

**7) C collaboration between health workers and traditional healers**

Do you collaborate with local traditional practitioners?

/__/ Yes /__/ No

If so, in what cases?

In your opinion, what are the reasons for refusing to collaborate?

/__/ lack of confidence /__/ Protection of endogenous knowledge

/__/ Inefficiency /__/ Poor quality of care and products

/__/ Fear of competition /__/ Inferiority complex

Do you ever refer patients to traditional practitioners?

/__/ Yes /__/ No /__/ Rare times

How can we correct this refusal to cooperate?

/__/ through dialogue /__/ through cross-fertilization /__/ through training /__/

**8) Reception in health centers**

Did you know that healthcare workers are generally criticized for their lack of enthusiasm in welcoming patients?

/__/ Yes /__/ No

Are you also criticized for the high cost of your services?

/_/ YES /__/ No

**9) Visits to health centers**

What is your center's attendance rate in relation to the local population?

/__/ Between 0- 5% /__/ 5-10% /__/ 10-20% /__/ More than 20% /__/ Between 0- 5% /__/ 5-10% /__/ 10-20% /__/ More than 20

Compared to traditional medicine?

/__/ Higher /__/ Lower /__/ Equal

What do you think are the real reasons for this discrepancy?

/__/ Cost of treatment /__/ Distance from health centers

/__/ Patient reception /__/ doesn't trust modern medicine
__ //Other ........................................................to be specified

**10) Training school**

Can the creation of a training school for Traditional Medicine in Benin contribute to improving the environment in which Traditional Medicine is practiced, and if so, how?

/__/ Promote the establishment of a framework for exchange /__/ Encourage collaboration between players in the two types of medicine /__/ Create a framework for training and capacity-building for traditional medicine practitioners /__/ Respect WHO standards for the production of improved traditional medicines.

**11) Traditional medicines**

**What does the future hold for medicinal plants in Benin?**

/__/ uncertain /__/ Promising

**What do you think about the proliferation of Chinese medicine in Africa in general and in Benin in particular?**

/__/ Dangerous competition for the promotion of Beninese traditional medicine /__/ Helping local initiatives /__/ Inspiring African countries /__/ Compromising the development of the national pharmacopoeia

**12) INTEGRATING TRADITIONAL MEDICINE**

**What advice do you have for traditional practitioners and scientists on how to achieve the goal of integrating Traditional Medicine into Benin's healthcare system?**

/__/ collaboration /__ / complementarity /_ / working in a vacuum

**NB: Multiple answers are allowed in this survey.**

SURVEY OF COMMUNITY KNOWLEDGE, ATTITUDES AND PRACTICES RELATED TO TRADITIONAL MEDICINE

**IV- Discussion guide for third parties**

Meeting place : ...........................................................................................

Number of participants :..........................................................................

The gender approach is widely shared and taken into account by our groups

**Level of information on Traditional Medicine.**

/__/ Sufficient

/__ / Insufficient

/__/ Approximate

**1- Experience in the use of traditional medicine**

/__ / Long

/__/ Short

/__/ Inexistent

**2- What do you appreciate about Traditional Medicine?**

/__/ Efficient methods

/__/ treatment efficacy

/__ / Treatment durability

/__/ Lower treatment costs

/__/ The holistic nature of this treatment method

**3- What's wrong with this kind of medicine?**

/__/ The lie

/__/ Unhealthy practices

/__ / Breach of trust

/__/ Obscurantism

/__/ Quackery

/__/ Lack of expertise in disease management techniques, particularly for chronic illnesses

/__/ Non-compliance with medical standards

**4- How would you like to see a mixed healthcare center set up in your community?**

/__/ Good

/__/ Bad

/__/ No opinion

**5- What do you think Benin can learn from its traditional medicine?**

/__/ Increasing access to primary healthcare

/__/ Serve as an alternative medicine

/__/ Promote the country's economic and social development.

/__/ Promoting the local industry for the production of safe traditional medicines

**6- What do you think is holding up the integration of traditional medicine into Benin's healthcare system?**

/__/ Lack of justification of scientific evidence

/__/ Lack of collaboration between health workers and traditional practitioners

/__/ Insufficient or no funding for scientific research

/__/ Inadequate qualification of traditional practitioners in disease management.

/__/ Lack of an appropriate legislative, regulatory and institutional framework

**7- How do you see the future of Benin's main pharmacopoeia resources, particularly plant resources?**

/__/ Uncertain

/__/ Reassured

/__/ Precarious

**8- What threats and pressures jeopardize this future?**

/__/ Logging

/__/ Bush fires

/__/ Climate change

/__/ Growing methods

**9- What are the best strategies for ensuring the long-term future of medicinal plants?**

/__/ Empowering plant sources through the spread of botanical gardens

/__/ Protecting rare plant species

/__/ Promoting medicinal plant exports

in Benin.

**How can we ensure the protection of traditional knowledge and know-how?**

/ __/ Strengthening national legislation

/__/ popularizing intellectual property law

/Valorize traditional therapeutic knowledge by producing medicines from medicinal plants to facilitate their protection by patents.

**V-** INTERVIEW GUIDE FOR TRADITIONAL MEDICINE MERCHANTS

Survey date :

Survey area :

Department :

Municipality :

Borough :

Village/ City district :

Ethnic group :

Gender :

Age :

Level of education :

Occupation :

Religion:

Marital status :

1) How long have you been in the business?
2) how did you get into the business?
3) Do you belong to a family of traditional practitioners?
4) Do you ever deliver the wrong materials to your customers?
5) What are the sources of your supplies?
6) How do you store your materials?
7) Do you share the opinion that your business generates too much profit?
8) What are your price ranges?
9) Do you have any other activities?
10) How do you ensure your succession in the business?
11) Do you think this activity has any impact on biodiversity?
12) What safeguarding action do you recommend?

13) What is your annual turnover?

14) Do you belong to a trade union?

15) Is there a union in your corporation?

16) Do you have export markets for your materials outside Benin? If so, which ones?

# BIBLIOGRAPHY


## 1- General books and documents

- ADJANAHOUN (E.) et al. 1986. Contribution aux études ethnobotanique et floristiques au Bénin. Paris, ACCT, Ed.
- Commune d'Agbangnizoun, 2004- 2008. Commune Development Plan (PDC), pp 27.
- Commune de Kétou, 2004. Plan de développement de la commune (PDC), Tome I, pp 56.
- Commune de Nikki, 2005. Plan de développement de la commune(PDC), pp 45.
- Commune de Savè, 2006. Rapport du schéma directeur d'aménagement de la commune, pp Cité pp 66.
- INSAE, 2002. Recensement Général de la Population et des Habitats (RGPH),
- KEREKOU(M), 1972. Discours programme du 30 Novembre 1972, Cotonou. 62pp
- KOUKPO (S. R.), 2002. Le droit à la santé au Bénin: Etat des lieux. Réseau des chercheurs " Droit à la santé " ; Agence Universitaire des statistiques sanitaires, MSP, Benin. Quoted by PETIT Pascale in: Histoire, enjeux et défis de l'intégration de la Médecine traditionnelle dans le système de santé en République du Bénin. Master2 thesis in health systems engineering, 2007.
- OUENDO (E.M), 2009. Sampling; research methodology seminar. Ecole doctorale pluridisciplinaire espace culture et développement (FLASH).Bénin, pp 27
- YARI (B. J.)2008. ODUDUA: Bref aperçu de l'origine des peuples Yoruba Soul edition - info Bénin, pp 25.

## 2 - Special Works and Documents

- Agence de Coopération Culturelle et Technique (ACCT), 1987. Traditional medicine and pharmacopoeia: bulletin de liaison. Paris. VOL 2; no 1, 129 p
- Astin (J.A.), 1993. Why patients use alternative medicine: Results of a national sturdy. Journal of the American medical association. Paris.
- Bannermann (R.B.), Buton (J) and Wen -Chieh (C.) 1983. " Traditional medicine and health care coverage,"
- International Development Research Centre (IDRC), 2004.13th International Conference on AIDS and Sexually Transmitted Diseases in Africa, Newsletter (WWW. WHO. Org)
- CONEJO (M.) ; ECOSOC/WHO 2009.Report on traditional medicine. Internal source: (WWW. OMS. Org)
- DALZIEL (J.M.), 1948. The useful plants of tropical West Africa. London. The Crown Agent for the Colonies. pp 19
- DANNERMANN (R.H.), 1982 Traditional medicine in modern health care, world health

Forum, 8- 13p
- Davy (M.) Cited by IDRC, 2001(W.W.W.OMS.Org)
- Décret no 86- 69 du 3 Mars 1986 portant statut et règlement intérieur de l'association nationale des praticiens de la médecine traditionnelle du Bénin, pp 26.
- ECOSOC, 2009. United Nations Economic and Social Council (www.OMS.org).
- GBEASSOR(M.), 2004. Reported by the International Development Research Centre (IDRC) (www.OMS.org).
- ***Houghton P.J., Raman A.*** *in Laboratory handbook for the fractionation of natural extracts. 1998, Chapman and Hall, London*
- Institut de formation sociale économique et civique and Friedrich NAUMANN Foundation, 1978. African pharmacopoeia and traditional medicine for the masses. Premier séminaire international. Cotonou pp 66.
- JAFFRE (Y.) and OLIVIER de SARDAN (J.P.), 2003. Une médecine inhospitalière: les difficiles relations entre soignants et soignés dans cinq capitales d'Afrique de l'Ouest. Paris, APAD- Karthala, p p462.
- KERHARO (J.) and BOUQUET (A.), 1980. Sorciers, Féticheurs et Guérisseurs de la Côte - d'Ivoire, Haute - Volta : Les hommes, les croyances, les pratiques, pharmacopée et thérapeutiques, p p 295.
- The global medicinal plant market, 2009 (http// www.who.net).
- MANDER (M.), 2009. Promoting the development of a modern industry based on the use of medicinal plants to design African products for African consumers, IDRC.
- Mason (F.) 1995. The complementary treatment project's treatment survey Toronto,
- Ministère Congolais et de la Population, 2006. Politique nationale de médecine traditionnelle, April, (www.OMS.org),
- MS/DPP/ SNIGS, 2002. Annuaire des statistiques sanitaires (Ministry of Health), pp 111
- OKPAKO (D.T.), 1999. Traditional African medicine: Theory and pharmacology explored Trends in Pharmacological Science Vol 20, pp 482-485.
- WHO, 2002, WHO Strategy for Traditional Medicine 2002-2005 WHO /EDM / TRM/, Geneva, pp 65
- WHO, 1976. African Traditional Medicine AFRO Regional Office Technical Report Series, - No. 1
- WHO, 2005. Promoting the role of traditional medicine in health systems: strategy for the African region,
- OUINSOU(S.E.), 1994. Traditional medicine: Conditions of emergence and fundamental features. The case of Africa and Benin in particular. Research work.
- (UN), 2009. Report of the round table on the contribution of traditional medicine to achieving international development goals related to global public health, (www.OMS.org)
- - African Intellectual Property Organization (OAPI), 2003. Référentiel pour l'Harmonisation des procédures d'homologation des médicaments issus de la pharmacopée

traditionnelle dans les pays membres de l'OAPI, pp 24.
- Ostrow (M.J.) et al, 1997. Determinants of complementary therapy use in HIV infected individuals receiving antiretroviral or anti opportunistic agents. Journal of acquired immune deficiency syndromes and human retrovirology.
- PAPE (O. N.), 2008. Sénégal santé, Agence Sénégalaise de Presse (ASP) November.
- PNPMT, 1965. Arrêté no 1146/ MSP/ DGM / DRMPT du 26 Mars1965 portant création de la direction de la recherche, de la médecine et de la pharmacopée traditionnelle
- PNPMT, 2008 Manuel d'initiation des agents de santé aux systèmes d'éducation et de transmission du savoir en médecine traditionnelle au Bénin. Cotonou
- PNPMT, 2009. STI and HIV/AIDS management protocol based on effective traditional practices in Benin. Cotonou
- PNPMT, 2009 - Traditional medicine; Newsletter No. 000, October.
- PNPMT, 2008. Manuel d'initiation des agents de santé aux systèmes d'éducation et de transmission de la médecine traditionnelle au Bénin. Cotonou.
- PNPMT, 2008. STI and HIV/AIDS management protocol based on effective traditional practices in Benin.
- PNPMT, 2009. Traditional medicine. 000 October Newsletter.
- PROMETRA - International, 2005. Pour une introduction judicieuse de la médecine traditionnelle dans les systèmes de santé nationaux du tiers monde, pp 2007.
- Resolution AFR/ RC50/R3, 2001. Concerning: Promoting the role of traditional medicine in health systems: strategy for the African region. WHO Regional Office for Africa, pp3
- ROSNY (E.)(de), 1992. L'Afrique des guérisons, Paris Karthala, 244 p.
- - SAYI (I.), 1978. Pharmacopée africaine et Médecine traditionnelle au service des masses populaires; Premier séminaire international. Cotonou, pp 13
- SOFOWORA. (A.), 1996. Plantes médicinales et Médecine traditionnelle d'Afrique, Karthala, Déc. pp 384.
- Studdert (D.M.) et al, 1998 Medical malpractice implications of alternative medicine. Journal of the American medical association.
- -TONDA (J.), 1988. "Healing power, healing and power in "outlaw" churches: an essay on the ideological production of the need for health," doc. Reno, 78 pp.
- VERGER (P), 1976.Tranquilliser and stimulants in Yoruba pharmaceutics; Institute of African studies, university of Ibadan,
- VERGER (P), (1976- 1977) The use of plants in Yoruba Traditional Medicine and its linguistic approach, department of African language and literatures, of Ifè, in seminar series, p-242- 295.
- VERGER (P.), 1997. EWE ; Le verbe et le pouvoir des plantes chez les Yoruba (Nigeria-Benin). Edition Maisonneuve et Larose, Paris, ISBN: 27068-1302-4, pp 730
- VERGER(P), 1976. Poisons and antidotes at the Language Department of the University of IFE, seminar.
- VERGER (P) and MING (A), 1990. Recherches sur les plantes à actions tonifiantes et stimulantes chez les Yoruba en Afrique et au Brésil. Published in Ethnopharmacologie:

Sources, méthodes, objectifs colloque et séminaires (colloque européen d'ethnopharmacologie, Metz, Mars1990). p.452- 453

- VERGER (P) and MING (A), 1993. Issoyé : Médications de la Mémoire chez les Yoruba en Afrique et au Brésil " ; Médicaments et aliments, approche Ethnopharmacologique, Paris, Orstom, p. 174- 177. (Cf.1993- Compte -rendu du 2[nd] Colloquium on Ethnopharmacology) (ESE) Heidelberg, March 24- 25, p p.49.

## 3 -Legal documents

- Arrêté 280/ MSP /DGM/DPH du 27 Janvier 1989 portant adoption d'une liste nationale de médicaments essentiels.
- Arrêté interministériel no 9960/ MSP/ DC / SGM/ DPED/C-P /MT/SA du 03 Novembre 2004, portant réglementation de la publicité en matière de la pharmacopée et médecine traditionnelles au Bénin, pp 3.
- Arrêté n° 1146/MSP/ DGM/DRMPT du 26 Mars 1965 : portant reconnaissance et promotion de la Médecine Traditionnelle au Dahomey.
- Law n° 93- 009 of July 2, 1993 on forest management in the Republic of Benin.
- Decree no. 96-271 of July 2, 1996 implementing the July 2 law
- Decree no. 86- 69 of March 3, 1986 on the statutes and internal regulations of the national association of traditional medicine practitioners of Benin.
- Decree no. 2001- 036 of February 15, 2001 establishing the principles of professional ethics and the conditions of practice of traditional medicine in the Republic of Benin.

## 4 - Theses and dissertations

- ALLAN (M.), 2008. Intégration de la médecine traditionnelle dans les systèmes de santé en Afrique : Cas du Bénin. Master 2 thesis in health economics, pp.56.
- HOUNIGNIHIN(R.A), 2005. Les mécanismes endogènes de prise en charge de l'ulcère de Buruli au Sud du Bénin. Doctoral thesis in environmental management and health. Cotonou, p p.248.
- NATABOU (D.F.), 1991. Contribution à l'étude de la médecine et pharmacopée traditionnelles au Bénin : Tentatives d'intégration dans le système de santé officiel. Thèse de doctorat en pharmacie, Dakar, p 135
- Olivier (de la. V.), 2001. Le concept de performance et sa mesure: Un état de l'art, pp. 21 CLAREE CNRS. Paris.
- PETIT (P.), 2007. Histoire, enjeux et défis de l'intégration de la Médecine traditionnelle dans le système de santé en République du Bénin. Master2 thesis in health systems engineering, Marseille, pp.45.

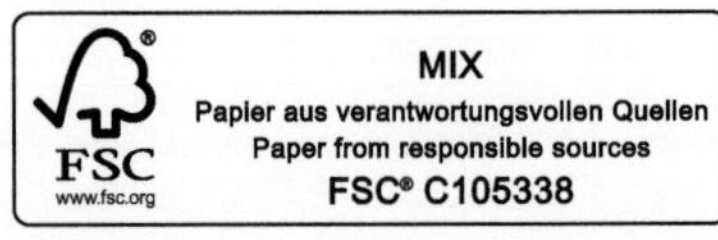


Printed by Books on Demand GmbH, Norderstedt / Germany